KETO FOR WOMEN

300 recipes

This Book Includes : "Keto Diet For Women Over 50 + Keto Diet for Beginners + Keto For Women After 50 "

Sara Clark

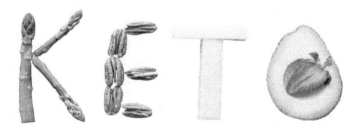

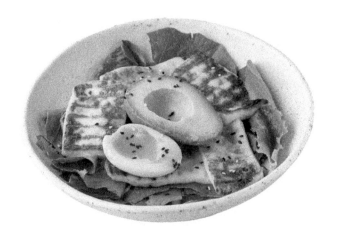

The trademarks used are without any consent, and the publication of the trademark is without permission or backing by the trademark owner. All trademarks and brands within this book are for clarifying purposes only and are owned by the owners themselves, not affiliated with this document.

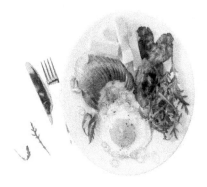

KETO DIET FOR WOMEN OVER 50

Contents

KETO DIET FOR BEGINNERS

Contents

KETO FOR WOMEN AFTER 50

Table of Contents

Chapter: 4 Meal keto recipes 244

Chapter 5: Drink recipes 254

Chapter 6: Vegetable Recipes 259

Chapter 10: Keto ice cream recipes and frozen treats 305

Conclusion 314

KETO DIET FOR WOMEN OVER 50

The Complete Ketogenic Diet Step by Step To Learn How to Easily Lose Weight for Woman

By Jason Smith

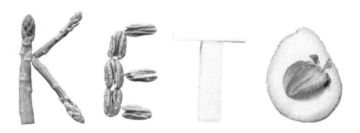

Introduction

The keto diet is a diet that has higher and lower fat values. It decreases glucose & insulin levels and changes the body's digestion away from carbohydrates and more towards fat & ketones. A word used in a low-carb diet is "Ketogenic." The concept is to provide more calories from fat and protein and few from sugars. The consumption of a high, low-sugar diet, adequate-protein, is used in medicine to achieve difficult (unstable) epilepsy control in young people. Instead of sugar, the diet allows the body to eat fats. Usually, the nutritious starches are converted to sugar, which will then be distributed throughout the body and is particularly important in filling the mind's work. Keto diet can cause enormous declines in the levels of glucose and insulin.

How food affects your body

Our metabolic procedures survive if we do not get the right details, and our well-being declines. We can get overweight, malnourished, and at risk for the worsening of diseases and disorders, such as inflammatory disease, diabetes, and cardiovascular disease if women get an unhealthy amount of essential nutrients or nourishment that provides their body with inadequate guidance. The dietary supplements allow the cells in our bodies to serve their essential capacities. This quote from a well-known workbook shows how dietary supplements are important for our physical work. Supplements are the nourishment feed substances necessary for the growth, development, and support of the body's capacities. Fundamental claimed that when a supplement is absent, capability sections and thus decrease in human health. The metabolic processes are delayed when the intake of supplements usually may not fulfill the cell activity's supplement requirements.

The keto diet involves keeping to a relatively low-carb, high-fat diet to put the body into a physiological state called ketosis. This makes fat intake increasingly productive for the health. When starting the diet, the ketogenic diet can induce a decrease in the drive, as the dieter will suffer side effects of carb removal and possibly low carb influenza. Whenever the detox and influenza-like symptoms have gone, and the dieter has transitioned to the reduced way of living, leading to weight loss from the diet, the charisma would in all likelihood reset and probably be comparable to earlier. Although the drive alert has a lot of credibility in the mainstream, in other words, supplementation provides advice to our bodies on how to function. In this sense, nourishment can be seen as a source of "information for the body." Pondering food along these lines gives one a view of the nourishment beyond calories or grams, fantastic food sources, or bad food sources. Instead of avoiding food sources, this perspective pushes us to reflect on the nutrients we can add. Instead of reviewing nourishment as the enemy, we look at nourishment to reduce health and disease by having the body look after ability.

Kidney and Heart Disease

When the body is low in electrolytes and fluid over the increased pee, electrolyte loss, such as magnesium, sodium, and potassium, can be caused. This will render people inclined to suffer serious kidney problems. Flushing out is not a joke and can lead to light-headedness, damage to the kidney, or kidney problems. Just like electrolytes are essential for the heart's standard stomping, this can place a dieter at the risk of cardiac arrhythmia. "Electrolyte appears to lack are not joking, and that may bring in an irregular heartbeat, that can be harmful,"

Yo-yo Dieting designs

When individuals encounter difficulties staying on the prohibitive diet indefinitely, the keto diet will also cause yo-yo dieting. That can have other adverse effects on the body.

Other effects

Other responses can involve terrible breath, fatigue, obstruction, irregular menstrual periods, reduced bone density, and trouble with rest. For even the most part, other consequences are not so much considered since it is impossible to observe dieters on a long-term assumption to discover the food schedule's permanent effects.

Wholesome Concerns

"There is still a dread amongst healthcare professionals that certain high intakes of extremely unhealthy fats will have a longer journey negative effect," she explained. Weight loss will also, for the time being, complicate the data. As overweight people get in form, paying less attention to how they do so, they sometimes end up with much better lipid profiles and blood glucose levels.

In comparison, the keto diet is extremely low in particular natural ingredients, fruits, nuts, and veggies that are as nutritious as a whole. Without these supplements, fiber, some carbohydrates, minerals, including phytochemicals that come along with these nourishments, will move through people on a diet. In the long run, this has vital public health consequences, such as bone degradation and increased risk of infinite diseases.

Sodium

The mixture of sodium (salt), fat, sugar, including bunches of sodium, will make inexpensive food more delicious for many people. However, diets rich in sodium will trigger fluid retention, which is why you can feel puffy, bloated, or swelled up in the aftermath of consuming cheap food. For those with pulse problems, a diet rich in sodium is also harmful. Sodium can increase circulatory stress and add weight to the cardiovascular structure. If one survey reveals, about % of grown-ups lose how much salt is in their affordable food meals. The study looked at 993 adults and found that the initial prediction was often smaller than the actual figure (1,292 mg). This suggests the sodium gauges in the abundance of 1,000 mg is off. One affordable meal could be worth a significant proportion of your day.

Impact on the Respiratory Framework

An overabundance of calories can contribute to weight gain from cheap foods. This will add to the weight. Obesity creates the risk of respiratory conditions, including asthma with shortness of breath. The extra pounds can put pressure on the heart and lungs, and with little intervention, side effects can occur. When you walk, climb stairs, or work out, you can notice trouble breathing. For youngsters, the possibility of respiratory problems is especially obvious. One research showed that young people who consume cheap food at least three days a week are bound to develop asthma.

Impact on the focal sensory system

For the time being, cheap food may satisfy hunger; however, long-haul effects are more detrimental. Individuals who consume inexpensive food and processed bakery items are

51 percent bound to generate depression than people who do not eat or eat either of those foods.

Impact on the conceptive framework

The fixings in cheap food and lousy nourishment can affect your money. One analysis showed that phthalates are present in prepared nourishment. Phthalates are synthetic compounds that can mess with the way your body's hormones function. Introduction to substantial amounts of these synthetics, like birth absconds, could prompt regenerative problems.

Impact on the integumentary framework (skin, hair, nails)

The food you eat may affect your skin's appearance, but it's not going to be the food you imagine. The responsibility for skin dry out breakouts has traditionally been claimed by sweets and sticky nourishments such as pizza. Nevertheless, as per the Mayo Clinic, there are starches. Carb-rich foods cause glucose jumps, and these sudden leaps in glucose levels can induce inflammation of the skin. Additionally, as shown by one investigation, young people and young women who consume inexpensive food at any pace three days a week are expected to create skin inflammation. Dermatitis is a skin disease that causes dry, irritated skin spots that are exacerbated.

Impact on the skeletal framework (bones)

Acids in the mouth can be enlarged by carbohydrates and sugar in inexpensive food and treated food. These acids may distinguish tooth lacquer. Microorganisms can take hold when the tooth veneer disappears, and depressions can occur. Weight will also prompt issues with bone thickness and bulk. The more severe chance of falling and breaking bones is for heavy individuals. It is important to continue training, develop muscles that support the bones, and sustain a balanced diet to prevent bone loss. One investigation showed that the measure of calories, sugar, and sodium in cheap food meals remains, to a large degree, constant because of attempts to bring problems to light and make women more intelligent consumers. As women get busier and eat out more often, it could have antagonistic effects on women and America's healthcare structure.

Chapter 1: Keto Diet and Its Benefits

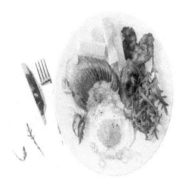

In the case of a ketogenic diet, the aim is to restrict carbohydrate intake to break down fat for power. When this occurs, to produce ketones that are by-products of the metabolism, the liver breaks down fat. These ketones are used in the absence of glucose to heat the body. A ketogenic diet takes the body into a "ketosis" mode. A metabolic condition that happens as ketone bodies in the blood contains most of the body's energy rather than glucose from carbohydrate-produced foods (such as grains, all sources of sugar or fruit). This compares with a glycolytic disorder, where blood glucose produces most of the body's power.

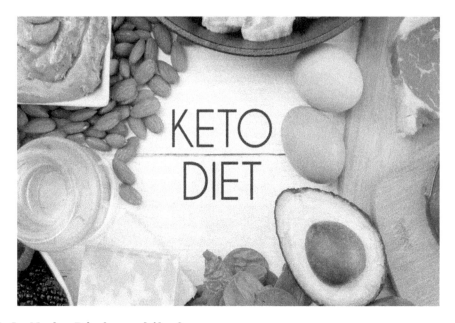

1.1. Keto Diet and its Success

The keto diet is successful in many studies, especially among obese men and women. The results suggest that KD can help manage situations such as:

- Obesity.
- Heart disease.

It is difficult to relate the ketogenic diet to cardiovascular disease risk factors. Several studies have shown that keto diets may contribute to substantial reductions in overall cholesterol, rises in levels of HDL cholesterol, decreases in levels of triglycerides and decreases in levels of LDL cholesterol, as well as possible changes in levels of blood pressure.

- Neurological disorders, including Alzheimer's, dementia, multiple sclerosis and Parkinson's.

- Polycystic ovarian syndrome (PCOS), among women of reproductive age, is the most prevalent endocrine condition.
- Certain forms of cancer, including cancers of the liver, colon, pancreas and ovaries.
- Diabetes Type 2. Among type 2 diabetics, it can also minimize the need for drugs.
- Seizure symptoms and seizures.
- And others.

•

1.2. Why Do the Ketogenic Diet

By exhausting the body from its sugar store, Ketogenic works to start sorting fat and protein for vitality, inducing ketosis (and weight loss).

1. Helps in weight loss

To convert fat into vitality, it takes more effort than it takes to turn carbohydrates into vitality. A ketogenic diet along these lines can help speed up weight loss. In comparison, because the diet is rich in protein, it doesn't leave you starving as most diets do. Five findings uncovered tremendous weight loss from a ketogenic diet in a meta-examination of 13 complex randomized controlled preliminaries.

2. Diminishes skin break out

There are different causes for the breakout of the skin, and food and glucose can be established. Eating a balanced diet of prepared and refined sugars can alter gut microorganisms and emphasize sensational variances in glucose, both of which would affect the skin's health. Therefore, that is anything but surprising that a keto diet may reduce a few instances of skin inflammation by decreasing carb entry.

3. May help diminish the danger of malignancy

There has been a lot of study on the ketogenic diet and how it could effectively forestall or even cure those malignant growths. One investigation showed that the ketogenic diet might be a corresponding effective treatment with chemotherapy and radiation in people with malignancy. It is because it can cause more oxidative concern than in ordinary cells in malignancy cells.

Some hypotheses indicate that it may decrease insulin entanglements, which could be linked to some cancers because the ketogenic diet lowers elevated glucose.

4. Improves heart health

There is some indication that the diet will boost cardiac health by lowering cholesterol by accessing the ketogenic diet in a balanced manner (which looks at avocados as a healthy fat rather than pork skins). One research showed that LDL ("Terrible") cholesterol levels fundamentally expanded among those adopting the keto diet. In turn, the LDL ("terrible") cholesterol fell.

5. May secure mind working

More study into the ketogenic diet and even the mind is needed. A few studies indicate that the keto diet has Neuro-protective effects. These can help treat or curtail Parkinson's, Alzheimer's, and even some rest problems. One research also showed that young people had increased and psychological work during a ketogenic diet.

6. Possibly lessens seizures

The theory that the combination of fat, protein, and carbohydrates modifies how vitality is utilized by the body, inducing ketosis. Ketosis is an abnormal level of Ketone in the blood. In people with epilepsy, ketosis will prompt a reduction in seizures.

7. Improves health in women with PCOS

An endocrine condition that induces augmented ovaries with pimples is polycystic ovarian disorder PCOS). On the opposite, a high-sugar diet can affect those with PCOS. On the ketogenic diet and PCOS, there are not many clinical tests. One pilot study involving five women on 24 weeks showed that the ketogenic diet:

- Aided hormone balance
- Improved luteinizing hormone (ILH)/follicle-invigorating hormone (FSH) proportions
- Increased weight loss
- Improved fasting insulin

For children who suffer the adverse effects of a particular problem (such as Lennox-gastaut disease or Rett disorder) and do not respond to seizure prescription, keto is also prescribed as suggested by the epilepsy foundation.

They note that the number of seizures these children had can be greatly reduced by keto, with 10 to 15 percent turns out to be sans seizure. It may also help patients to reduce the portion of their prescription in some circumstances. Be it as it can, the ketogenic diet still many effective trials to back up its advantages. For adults with epilepsy, the keto diet can likewise be helpful. It was considered as preferable to other diets in supporting people with:

- Epilepsy
- Type 2 diabetes
- Type 1 diabetes
- High blood pressure
- Heart disease
- Polycystic ovary syndrome
- Fatty liver disease
- Cancer
- Migraines

- Alzheimer's infection
- Parkinson's infection
- Chronic inflammation
- High blood sugar levels
- Obesity

The ketogenic diet will be beneficial, regardless of whether you are not in danger from any of these disorders. A portion of the advantages that are enjoyed by the vast majority are:

- An increment in vitality
- Improved body arrangement
- Better cerebrum work
- A decline in aggravation

As should be clear, the ketogenic diet has a vast variety of advantages, but is it preferable to other diets?

8. Treating epilepsy — the origins of the ketogenic diet

Until sometime in 1998, the major analysis on epilepsy and the keto diets was not distributed. Of about 150 children, almost each of whom had several seizures a week, despite taking two psychosis drugs in either situation. The children were given a one-year initial ketogenic diet. Around 34 percent of infants, or slightly more than 33 percent, had a 90 percent decline in seizures after three months.

The healthy diet was claimed to be "more feasible than just a substantial lot of new anticonvulsant medications and is much endured by families and kids when it is effective." Not only was the keto diet supportive. It was, however, more useful than other drugs usually used.

9. Improving blood pressure with the ketogenic diet

A low-sugar intake is more effective at reducing the pulse than just a low-fat or moderate-fat diet. Restricting starches often provides preferable results over the mix of a low-fat regimen and a relaxing weight-loss/pulse.

10. The power to improve Alzheimer's disease

Alzheimer's disease patients also agree with organic chemistry." high sugar acceptance deepens academic performance in patient populations with Alzheimer's infectious disease." It means that more starches are consumed in the cerebrum. Will the reverse (trying to eat fewer carbs) improve the functioning of the cerebrum?

Other mental health benefits that ketone bodies have:

- They forestall neuronal loss.
- They ensure synapses against various sorts of damage.
- They save neuron work.

•

1.3. The Benefits of Ketogenic Diet

The board provides many substantial advantages when choosing a ketogenic diet for diabetes. Living in a stable ketosis state causes a tremendous change in blood glucose regulation and weight loss. Other frequent advantages provided include:

- Improvements in insulin affectability
- Lower circulatory strain
- Usually enhancements in cholesterol levels.
- Reduced reliance on taking drugs

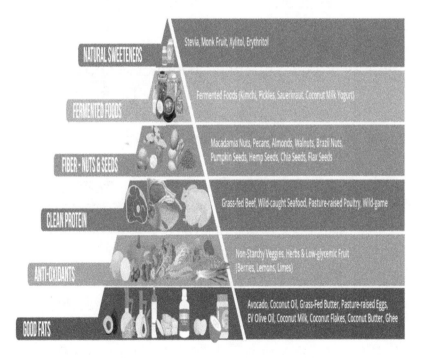

We send you a short science behind the ketogenic diet in this book and how it attempts to give these particular benefits.

1. Weight loss and support

The ketogenic diet's significant benefit is achieving accelerated weight loss, reducing starches necessary to be in a ketosis state, causing both a noteworthy decrease in muscle vs. fats and bulk increase and maintenance. Studies have shown that a low-carb, keto diet can produce an all-inclusive duration of solid weight loss. For one year, a big person had the opportunity to lose, by and large, 15 kilograms. It was 3 kg, which is more than the low-fat food used in the study carried out.

2. Blood glucose control

The other main reason for maintaining a ketogenic diet for people with diabetes is its ability to reduce and regulate glucose levels. The substitute (macronutrient) that improves glucose the most is starch. Since the keto diet is low in starch, the greater rises in glucose are dispensed with. Ketogenic diets prove that they are effective in reducing hba1c, a long-term blood glucose regulation percentage. A natural decrease of 17 mmol/mol (1.5 percent) in hba1c levels for persons with type 2 diabetes. People with other forms of diabetes, such as diabetes and LADA, can also expect to see a strong decline in glucose levels and increase control. Remember that if an increase in blood glucose regulation is sustained over different years, this will reduce intricacies. It is necessary to play it safe for those on insulin, or otherwise at risk of hypos, to avoid the incidence of hypos.

Decreasing drug reliance on diabetes. Since it is so effective at lowering glucose levels, the keto diet provides the added benefit of allowing people with type 2 diabetes to decrease their dependency on diabetes medication. Persons on insulin and other hypertension prescriptions (Sulphonylureas & Glinides, for example) may need to reduce their portions before initiating a ketogenic diet to avoid hypotension. For advice on this, contact your primary care provider.

3. Insulin affectability

To further restore insulin affectability, a ketogenic diet has emerged since it dispenses with the root driver of insulin obstruction, which is too high insulin levels in the bloodstream. This diet advances supported periods with low insulin since low carbohydrate levels indicate lower insulin levels. A high diet of starch resembles putting petroleum on the insulin obstruction fire. A more influential need for insulin is indicated by elevated sugar, and this aggravates insulin opposition. A ketogenic diet, by correlation, turns down insulin levels since fat is the least insulin-requiring macronutrient. In comparison, bringing the insulin levels down also helps with fat intake, provided that elevated insulin levels inhibit fat breakdown. The body will differentiate fat cells at the point that insulin levels decrease for several hours.

4. Hypertension control

It is estimated that 16 million people in the U.K. suffer from hypertension. Hypertension, for example, cardiovascular disease, stroke, and renal disease, is related to the scope of health disorders. Different studies have demonstrated that a ketogenic diet can reduce circulatory stress levels in overweight or type 2 diabetes people. It is also a part of metabolic imbalance.

5. Cholesterol levels

For the most part, ketogenic diets bring in reductions in cholesterol levels. LDL cholesterol levels are usually reduced, and HDL cholesterol levels increase, which is healthy. The amount of absolute cholesterol to HDL is possibly the most substantiated proportion of safe cholesterol. It can be effectively detected by taking the full cholesterol result and partitioning it by your HDLS result. It indicates good cholesterol, on the off chance that the amount you get is 3.5 or lower. Study findings suggest that ketogenic diets are normally possible to increase this proportion of good cholesterol.

After starting a ketogenic, a few individuals can display an expansion in LDL and all-out cholesterol. It is generally taken as a bad indicator, but this does not speak of compounding in heart health if the absolute cholesterol to HDL ratio is appropriate.

Cholesterol is a confounding topic, and if your cholesterol levels essentially shift on a ketogenic diet, your PCP is the optimization technique of exhortation. More simple mental results. Other typically announced advantages of eating a ketogenic diet are emotional insight, an increased capacity to center, and superior memory. Expanding the admission of omega-3 healthy fats, such as those present in slick fish such as salmon, fish, and mackerel, will boost the state of mind and the ability to read. It is because omega-3 extends an unsaturated fat called DHAS, which makes up 15 to 30 percent of the cerebrum of females. The discovery of beta-hydroxybutyrate, a type of Ketone, allows for long-term memory work to be facilitated.

6. Satiety

The effects of ketogenic diets impact malnutrition. As the body responds to being in a ketosis state, it becomes acclimatized to obtain vitality from muscle to fat ratio differentiation, which will alleviate appetite and desires.

They are possible at:

- **Reducing desires**
- **Reducing inclination for sugary nourishments**
- **Helping you feel full for more**

Weight loss will also reduce leptin levels attributable to a ketogenic diet, which will increase the affectability of leptin and thus gain satiety.

1.4. Keto Shopping List

A keto diet meal schedule for women above 5o+ years and a menu that will transform the body. Generally speaking, the keto diet is low in carbohydrates, high in fat and moderate in protein. While adopting a ketogenic diet, carbs are routinely reduced to under 50 grams every day, but stricter and looser adaptations of the diet exist.

• Proteins can symbolize about 20 percent of strength requirements, whereas carbohydrates are usually restricted to 5 percent.

• The body retains its fat for the body to use as energy production.

Most of the cut carbs should be supplanted by fats and convey about 75% of your all-out caloric intake.

The body processes ketones while it is in ketosis, particles released from cholesterol in the blood glucose is low, as yet another source of energy.

Because fat is always kept a strategic distance from its unhealthy content, research demonstrates that the keto diet is essentially better than low-fat diets to advance weight reduction.

In contrast, keto diets minimize desire and improve satiation, which is especially useful when getting in shape.

Fatty cuts of PROTEIN: *Keto Diet Shopping list*
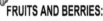

NUTS AND SEEDS:
1. MACADAMIA NUTS+BUTTER
2. BRAZIL NUTS+BUTTER
3. PECANS+BUTTER
4. WALNUTS
5. PUMPKIN SEEDS
6. ALMONDS +BUTTER

1. GROUND BEEF - RIBEYE STEAK
2. PORK BELLY ROAST +BACON
3. BEEF OR PORK SAUSAGE
4. WILD CAUGHT SALMON
5. SARDINES OR TUNA
6. CHICKEN THIGHS OR LEGS
7. TURKEY LEGS
8. DEER STEAKS
9. EGGS
10. DUCK EGGS
11.

Green Leafy VEGGIES:
1. BROCCOLI
2. CAULIFLOWER
3. GREEN BEANS
4. BRUSSEL SPROUTS
5. KALE
6. SPINACH
7. CHARD
8. CABBAGE
9. BOK CHOY
10. CELERY
11. ARUGULA
12. ASPARAGUS
13. ZUCCHINI
14. YELLOW SQUASH
15. MUSHROOMS
16. OLIVES
17. ARTICHOKE
18. CUCUMBERS
19. ONIONS
20. GARLIC
21. OKRA

FRUITS AND BERRIES:
1. POMEGRANATE
2. GRAPEFRUIT
3. BLUEBERRIES
4. RASPBERRIES
5. LEMON
6. LIME
7. AVOCADO

FATS:
1. BUTTER
2. OLIVE OIL
3. COCONUT OIL
4. COCONUT BUTTER
5. MCT OIL
6. AVOCADO
7. GHEE
8. BACON GREASE
9. AVOCADO OIL

MUST HAVE MISCELLANEOUS:
1. ALMOND+COCONUT FLOUR
2. COCONUT BUTTER
3. 85% DARK CHOCOLATE
4. PORK RINDS
5. COCONUT CREAM
6. COCONUT FLAKES

1.5. Keto-Friendly Foods to Eat

Meals and bites should be based on the accompanying nourishment when following a ketogenic diet:

Eggs: pastured eggs are the best choice for all-natural eggs.

Meat: hamburger grass- nourished, venison, pork, organ meat, and buffalo.

Full-fat dairy: yogurt, cream and margarine.

Full-fat Cheddar: Cheddar, mozzarella, brie, cheddar goat and cheddar cream.

Nuts and seeds: almonds, pecans, macadamia nuts, peanuts, pumpkin seeds, and flaxseeds.

Poultry: turkey and chicken.

Fatty fish: Wild-got salmon, herring, and mackerel

Nut margarine: Natural nut, almond, and cashew spreads.

Vegetables that are not boring: greens, broccoli, onions, mushrooms, and peppers.

Condiments: salt, pepper, lemon juice, vinegar, flavors and crisp herbs.

Fats: coconut oil, olive oil, coconut margarine, avocado oil, and sesame oil.

Avocados: it is possible to add whole avocados to practically any feast or bite.

1.6. Nourishments to avoid

Although adopting a keto diet, keep away from carbohydrate-rich nutrients.

It is important to restrict the accompanying nourishments:

- **Sweetened beverages:** beer, juice, better teas, and drinks for sports.
- **Pasta:** noodles and spaghetti.
- **Grains and vegetable articles:** maize, rice, peas, oats for breakfast
- **Starchy vegetables:** Butternut squash, Potatoes, beans, sweet potatoes, pumpkin and peas.
- **Beans and vegetables:** chickpeas, black beans, kidney beans and lentils.
- **Fruit:** citrus, apples, pineapple and bananas.
- **Sauces containing high-carbohydrates:** BBQ' sauce, a sugar dressing with mixed greens, and dipping's.
- **Hot and bread items:** white bread, whole wheat bread, wafers, cookies, doughnuts, rolls, etc.
- **Sweets and sweet foods:** honey, ice milk, candy, chocolate syrup, agave syrup, coconut sugar.
- **Blended refreshments:** Sugar-blended cocktails and beer.

About the assumption that carbs should be small, low-glycemic organic goods, for example, when a keto-macronutrient is served, spread, berries may be satisfied with restricted quantities. Be sure to choose safe sources of protein and eliminate prepared sources of food and bad fats.

It is worth keeping the accompanying stuff away from:

1. **Diet nutrients:** Foods containing counterfeit hues, contaminants and carbohydrates, such as aspartame and sugar alcohols.

2. **Unhealthy fats:** Such as corn and canola oil, include shortening, margarine, and cooking oils.

3. **Processed foods:** Fast foods, bundled food sources, and frozen meats, such as wieners and meats for lunch.

1.8. One week Keto Diet Plan

(Day 1): Monday

Breakfast: Eggs fried in seasoned butter served over vegetables.

Lunch: A burger of grass-bolstered with avocado, mushrooms, and cheddar on a tray of vegetables.

Dinner: Pork chops and French beans sautéed in vegetable oil.

(Day 2): Tuesday

Breakfast: Omelet of mushroom.

Lunch: Salmon, blended vegetables, tomato, and celery on greens.

Dinner: Roast chicken and sautéed cauliflower.

(Day 3): Wednesday

Breakfast: Cheddar cheese, eggs, and bell peppers.

Lunch: Blended veggies with hard-bubbled eggs, avocado, turkey, and cheddar.

Dinner: Fried salmon sautéed in coconut oil.

(Day 4): Thursday

Breakfast: Granola with bested full-fat yogurt.

Lunch: Steak bowl of cheddar, cauliflower rice, basil, avocado, as well as salsa.

Dinner: Bison steak and mushy cauliflower.

(Day 5): Friday

Breakfast: Pontoons of Avocado egg (baked).

Lunch: Chicken served with Caesar salad.

Dinner: Pork, with veggies.

(Day 6): Saturday

Breakfast: Avocado and cheddar with cauliflower.

Lunch: Bunless burgers of salmon.

Dinner: Parmesan cheddar with noodles topped with meatballs.

(Day 7): Sunday

Breakfast: Almond Milk, pecans and Chia pudding.

Lunch: Cobb salad made of vegetables, hard-boiled eggs, mango, cheddar, and turkey.

Dinner: Curry chicken.

Chapter 2: Health Concerns for Women Over 50+

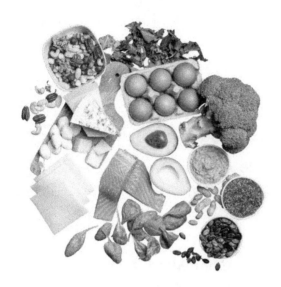

This chapter will give you a detailed view of the health concerns for women over 50.

2.1. Menopause

Healthy maturation includes large propensities such as eating healthy, avoiding regular prescription mistakes, monitoring health conditions, receiving suggested screenings, or being dynamic. Getting more seasoned involves change, both negative and positive, but you can admire maturing on the off chance of understanding your body's new things and finding a way to maintain your health. As you age, a wide range of things happens to your body. Unexpectedly, your skin, bones, and even cerebrum may start to carry on. Try not to let the advances that accompany adulthood get you off guard.

Here's a segment of the normal ones:

1. The Bones: In mature age, bones may become slender and progressively weaker, especially in women, leading to the delicate bone disease known as osteoporosis once in a while. Diminishing bones and decreasing bone mass can put you at risk for falls that can occur in broken bones without much of a stretch result. Make sure you talk to your doctor about what you can do to prevent falls and osteoporosis.

2. The Heart: While a healthy diet and normal exercise can keep your heart healthy, it may turn out to be somewhat amplified, lowering your pulse and thickening the heart dividers.

3. The Sensory system and Mind: It can trigger changes in your reflexes and even your skills by becoming more seasoned. While dementia is certainly not an ordinary outcome of mature age, individuals must encounter some slight memory loss as they become more stated. The formation of plaques and tangles, abnormalities that could ultimately lead to dementia, can harm cells in the cerebrum and nerves.

4. The Stomach: A structure associated with your stomach. As you age, it turns out that your stomach-related is all the more firm and inflexible and does not contract as often. For example, stomach torment, obstruction, and feelings of nausea can prompt problems with this change; a superior diet can help.

5. The Abilities: You can see that your hearing and vision is not as good as it ever was. Maybe you'll start losing your sense of taste. Flavors might not appear as unique to you. Your odor and expertise in touch can also weaken. In order to respond, the body requires more time and needs more to revitalize it.

6. The Teeth: Throughout the years, the intense veneer protecting your teeth from rot will begin to erode, making you exposed to pits. Likewise, gum injury is a problem for more developed adults. Your teeth and gums will guarantee great dental cleanliness. Dry mouth, which is a common symptom of seniors' multiple drugs, can also be a concern.

7. The Skin: Your skin loses its versatility at a mature age and can tend to droop and wrinkle. Nonetheless, the more you covered your skin when you were younger from sun exposure and smoke, the healthier your skin would look as you get more mature. Start securing your skin right now to prevent more injury, much like skin malignancy.

8. The Sexual Conviviality: When the monthly period ends following menopause, many women undergo physical changes such as vaginal oil loss. Men can endure erectile brokenness. Fortunately, it is possible to handle the two problems successfully.

A normal part of maturing is a series of substantial improvements, but they don't need to back you up. Furthermore, you should do a lot to protect your body and keep it as stable as you would imagine, given the circumstances.

2.2. Keys to Aging Well

Although good maturation must preserve your physical fitness, it is also vital to appreciate the maturity and growth you acquire with propelling years. Its fine to rehearse healthy propensities for an extraordinary period, but it's never beyond the point of no return to gain the benefits of taking great account of yourself, even as you get more developed.

Here are some healthy maturing tips at every point of life that are a word of wisdom:

- Keep dynamic physically with a normal workout.
- With loved ones and inside your locale, remain socially diverse.
- Eat a balanced, well-adjusted diet, dumping low-quality food to intake low-fat, fiber-rich, and low-cholesterol.
- Do not forget yourself: daily enrollment at this stage with your primary care provider, dental surgeon, and optometrist is becoming increasingly relevant.
- Taking all medications as the primary care provider coordinates.
- Limit the consumption of liquor and break off smoke.
- Receive the rest your body wants.

Finally, it is necessary to deal with your physical self for a long time, but it is vital that you still have an eye on your passionate health. Receive and enjoy the rewards of your long life every single day. It is the perfect chance to enjoy better health and pleasure.

1. Eat a healthy diet

For more developed development, excellent nourishment and sanitation are especially critical. You need to regularly ensure that you eat a balanced, tailored diet. To help you decide on astute diet options and practice healthy nutrition, follow these guidelines.

2. Stay away from common medication mistakes

Drugs can cure health conditions and allow you to continue to lead a long, stable life. Drugs may also cause real health problems at the stage that they are misused. To help you decide on keen decisions about the remedy and over-the-counter medications you take, use these assets.

3. Oversee health conditions

Working with your healthcare provider to monitor health issues such as diabetes, osteoporosis, and hypertension is important. To treat these regular health problems, you need to get familiar with the medications and gadgets used.

4. Get screened

Health scans are an effective means of helping to perceive health conditions - even before any signs or side effects are given. Tell the healthcare provider what direct health scans are for you to determine how much you can be screened.

5. Be active

Exercise, as well as physical action, can help you to remain solid and fit. You just don't have to go to an exercise center. Converse about proper ways that you really can be dynamic with your healthcare professional. Look at the assets of the FDA and our accomplices in the administration.

2.3. Skin Sagging

There are also ways to prevent age from sagging, which are:

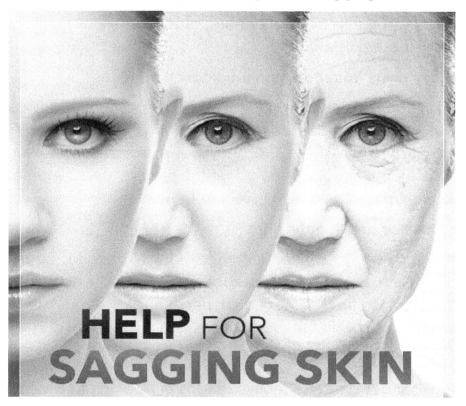

1. Unassuming Fixing and Lifting

These systems are called non-obtrusive methodologies of non-intrusive skin fixing on the basis that they leave your skin unblemished. A while later, you won't have a cut injury, a cut, or crude skin. You may see and grow some impermanent redness, but that is usually the main sign that you have a technique.

It is what you can expect from a skin-fixing method that is non-intrusive:

- **Results:** seem to come step by step, so they seem normal to be

- **Downtime:** zero to little

- **Colorblind:** secure for people with all skin hues

- **Body-wide use:** you can patch the skin almost anywhere on your body.

<u>Ultrasonic dermatologists use ultrasound to transmit heat deep into the tissue.</u>

Key concern: warming will induce more collagen to be created by your body. Many individuals see the unobtrusive raising and fixing within two and a half years of one procedure. By getting additional drugs, you can get more benefits.

<u>During this procedure, the dermatologist places a radiofrequency device on the skin that warms the tissue beneath.</u>

Key concern: Most people get one treatment and instantly feel an obsession. Your body needs some money to manufacture collagen, so you'll see the best effects in about half a year. By getting more than one treatment, a few persons benefit.

<u>Some lasers will send heat deeply through the skin without injuring the skin's top layer by laser therapy. These lasers are used to repair skin everywhere and can be especially effective for fixing free skin on the tummy and upper arms.</u>

Primary concern: to get outcomes, you may need 3 to 5 drugs, which occur step by step somewhere in the region of 2 and a half years after the last procedure.

2. Most fixing and lifting without medical procedure

While these methodologies will deliver you increasingly measurable results, considering all, they will not give you the aftereffects of an operation such as a facelift, eyelid surgical treatment, or neck lift, insignificantly pleasing to the eye skin fixing techniques. Negligibly obtrusive skin fixing requires less personal time than surgical treatment, however. It also conveys less chance of reactions.

3. How to look younger than your age without Botox, lasers and surgery, plus natural remedies for skin sagging

It is possible to become more experienced in this lifetime. However, you don't need to look at your age on the off chance you'd like not to. Truth be told, if you have been wondering how you would look as youthful as you feel, we will be eager to bet that you feel a lot more youthful than the amount you call your "age!"

2.4. Weight loss

Quality preparation builds the quality of your muscles and improves your versatility.

Even though cardio is very important for lung health and the heart, getting more fit and keeping it off is anything but an incredible technique.

The weight will return quickly at the point when you quit doing a lot of cardio. An unquestionable requirement has cardio as a component of your general wellness routine; be that as it may, when you start going to the exercise centre, quality preparation should be the primary factor. Quality preparation increases your muscle's quality, but this will enhance your portability and the main thing known to build bone thickness (alongside appropriate supplements).

Weight-bearing exercises help build and maintain bulk and build bone quality and reduce the risk of osteoporosis. Many people over [the age of] 50 will stop regularly practicing due to torment in their joints or back or damage, but do not surrender. In any case, understand that because of age-related illness, hormone changes, and even social variables such as a busy life, it may seem more enthusiastic to pick up muscle as you age. As he would like to think that to build durable muscles, cardio will consume off fat and pick substantial weights with few representatives or lighter weights. Similarly, for generally speaking health and quality, remember exercise and diet are linked to the hip, likewise, as the trick of the year. ! Locate a professional who can help you get back into the groove and expect to get 2 hrs. Thirty minutes of physical movement in any case [in] seven days to help to maintain your bulk and weight.

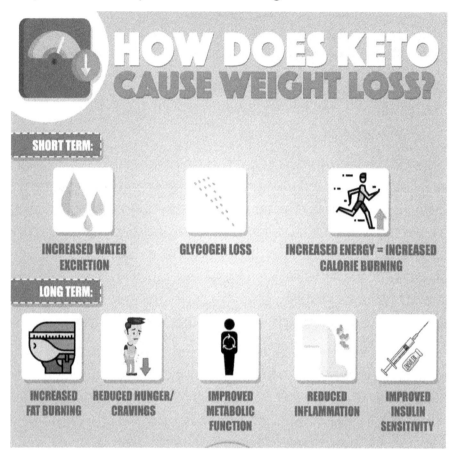

1. Try not to skip meals.

Testosterone and Estrogen decline gradually after some time, which also prompts fat collection because the body does not prepare sugar. We alternatively keep losing more bulk as we get older; this will cause our bodies' metabolic needs to lessen. Be that as it may, meal skipping can make you lack significant key medications required as we age, for example, by before large protein and calories. Tracking your energy levels throughout the day and obtaining sufficient calories/protein would also help you feel better on the scale, explaining how you will be burning more calories but less inefficiently. We also lose more bulk as we age, causing our metabolic rate to decrease. Be that as it may, skipping meals can make you lack important key supplements required as we age, for example, by an aging, metabolic rate.

2. Ensure you are getting enough rest.

"Perhaps the highest argument of over 50 years is a lack of rest," Amselem notes. Basically, rest may interfere with an important medical procedure, causing metabolic breakage in the system, in which the body turns weakness into hunger, urging you to eat. I plan to rest for seven to eight hours and, if necessary, take low rest. Rest is vital to a healthy weight because two hormones, leptin, and Ghrelin are released during rest, and they conclude a significant job in eating guidelines.

3. Relinquish old "rules" about weight loss and develop an outlook on health.

For the two women and men, age impacts weight loss, and that is on the basis that digestion backs off, hormone levels decay, in addition to there is a loss of bulk," "Nevertheless, that does not imply that mission is inconceivable to get more fit over age 50. Everybody else has to take a half hour's exercise, but there are two big reasons why it can't be done: you eat too much, or you are not active enough. The wellness movement encourages people to be aware of their own health, body and well-being. Being over 50 years old is not the end of the world. In fact, there is still a chance for us to live the rest of our lives as retirees. It is important to eat well, exercise, not smoke, and limit alcohol consumption in our lives. Our bodies are naturally aging, but we do not yet have to quit. Instead of falling prey to craze diets, make ongoing acclimatization to advance adjusted eating, and help yourself remember the benefits of exercise for your heart, stomach-related tract, and psychological well-being, despite the executives' weight.

2.5. Factors Influencing Fuel Utilization

The amount of each element in one's blood plasma determines the combination of fuels in the body. According to the researchers, the main element that determines how much of each nutrient is absorbed is the quantity of each nutrient eaten first by the body. The second considerations to take into account when assessing one's health is the amounts of hormones like insulin and glucagon, which must be in balance with one's diet. The third is the body's physical accumulation (cellular) of any nutrient, such as fat, muscle, and liver glycogen. Finally, the quantities of regulatory enzymes for glucose & fat breakdown beyond our influence, but changes in diet and exercise decide each gasoline's overall usage. Surely, both of these considerations will be discussed more extensively below.

1. Quantity of nutrients consumed

Humans will obtain four calories from sources in their surroundings: carbon, hydrogen, nitrogen, and oxygen. When it comes to the body demanding and using a given energy supply, it prefers to choose the nearest one to it due to the quantity and concentration in the bloodstream. The body can improve its use of glucose or decrease its use of glucose directly due to the amount of carbohydrate intake being ingested. It is an effort by the liver to control glycogen (sugar) levels in the body. If carbohydrate (carb) intake goes up, the use of carbohydrate-containing goods will go up, in exchange. Proteins are slightly harder to control. As protein consumption goes up, our bodies increase their development and oxidation of proteins as well. The food source for our body is protein. If it is in short supply, our body will consume less of it. This is an attempt to keep body protein cellular levels stable at 24-hour intervals. Since dietary fat does not lift the amount of fat the body needs, it cannot dramatically change how much fuel the body gets from that fat. Rather than measuring insulin directly, it is important to measure insulin indirectly, so it does not drift.

The blood alcohol content can decrease the body's energy reserves with those calories of fat. This will almost entirely impair the body's usage of fat for food. As most people know, carbohydrate intake will influence the amount of fat the body uses as a fuel supply. High carb diets increase the body's use of fat for food and the insulin threshold and amount. Therefore, the highest fat oxidation rates occur when there are low levels of carbohydrates in the body. Another clarification of this can be found in chapter 18, where it is clarified that the amount of glycogen regulates how much fat is used by the muscles. When a human eats less energy and carbohydrates, the body can subsequently take up fat calories for food instead of carbohydrates.

2. Hormone levels

Factors like food, exercise, medications and hormones all play a part in how we use our bodies' fuel. The hormone known as insulin is of high interest to many physicians because it plays a significant role in a wide range of activities, including the bodies functioning. A glance at the hormones involved in fuel consumption is included in the following passage.

Insulin is a peptide (as in the "peptide" in "peptides" that are essential in digestion) that the pancreas releases in response to changes in blood glucose. As blood glucose goes up, insulin levels also rise, and the body will use this extra glucose to kind of store it as glycogen in the muscles or in the liver. Glucose and extra glucose will be forced into fat cells for preservation (as alpha-glycerophosphate). Protein synthesis is enhanced, and as a result, amino acids (the building blocks of proteins) are transferred out of the blood via muscle cells and are then placed together to make bigger proteins. Fat synthesis or "lipogenesis" (making fat) and fat accumulation are also induced. In effect, it's hard for insulin to be released from fat cells due to even tiny levels of it. The main objective of insulin is regulating blood glucose in a very small range of around 80 to 120 milligrams per decilitre. When blood glucose levels rise outside of the normal range, insulin is released to get the glucose levels back into a normal range. The greatest rise in blood glucose levels (and the greatest increase in insulin) happens when humans eat carbohydrates in the diet. Due to amino acids that can be converted to glycogen, the breakdown of proteins can cause an increase the amount of insulin released. FFA can induce insulin release and produce ketone bodies found at concentrations that are far smaller than those produced by carbohydrates or proteins.

When your glucose level decreases, as it does with exercise and from eating less carbohydrate, your insulin levels decrease as well. During cycles with low insulin and higher hormones, the body's storage fuels can burst, leading to a breakdown of stored fuels. After accumulation within the body, triglycerides are broken down into fatty acids and glycerol and released into the bloodstream. Specific proteins might be broken down into individual amino acids and used as sources of sources glucose. Glycogen is a material contained in the liver that is broken when insulin is absent. Failure to produce insulin suggests a pathological state. Type me, diabetes (or Insulin Dependent Diabetes Mellitus, IDDM). In a group of patients with Type I diabetes (1), these patients have a deficiency in the pancreas, causing them to be entire without insulin. I already told you that to practical control glucose levels, people with diabetes have to inject themselves with insulin. This is relevant in the next chapter since the difference between diabetic ketoacidosis and dietary mediated ketosis is made in the chapter after this. Glucagon is essentially known as insulin's mirror hormone in the body and has nearly opposite effects. The enzyme insulin is also a peptide hormone made by the pancreas, which is released from the cells of the body, and its primary function as well is to sustain stable glucose levels. However, once blood glucose goes down below average, glucagon increases blood glucose on its own. The precursors are expelled from the cells into the bloodstream.

Glucagon's key function is in the liver, where it signals the degradation of liver glycogen and the resulting release into the bloodstream. The release of glucagon is modulated by what we eat, the sort of workout, and the presence of a meal that activates the development of glucagon in the body (24). High amounts of insulin suppress the pancreas from releasing the hormone glucagon. Normally, glucagon's actions are restricted to the liver; by comparison, its function in these other tissues is yet to be detected (i.e., fat and muscle cells). On the other hand, when insulin levels are very low, such as when glucose restriction and activity occur, glucagon plays a minor role in fat mobilization, as well as the degradation of muscle glycogen. Glucagon's primary function is to regulate blood glucose under conditions of low blood sugar. But it also plays a crucial role in ketone body development in the liver, which we will address in-depth in the next chapter. Below are the definitions of two contrasting hormones. It should be obvious from reading the sentences that they have opposite effects on one another. Whereas insulin is a key storage hormone that allows for the retention of accumulated glucose, potassium, albumin and fat in the body, glucagon serves the same role by allowing for the utilization of stored fat in an organism.

Insulin and glucagon are central to the determination to be anabolic or catabolic. However, their presence in the body is not alone enough for muscle development. Other hormones are involved as well. They will briefly be discussed below. Growth hormone, which is a peptide hormone, elicits various effects on the body, such as its effects on blood flow and muscle tissue growth. The hormone to hold appetite at bay, Ghrelin, is released in response to several stressors. Most notably, exercise, a reduction in blood glucose, and carbohydrate restriction or fasting can both induce Ghrelin production. As its name suggests (GH), GH is a growth-promoting hormone, which enhances protein production (protein synthesis) in the body and liver. Glucose, glycogen, and triglycerides also are mobilized from fat cells for nutrition.

Adrenaline and noradrenaline (also called epinephrine and norepinephrine) are members of a special family of hormones called 'fight or flight' hormones. They tend to be released in response to discomfort, such as running, fasting, or consuming cold foods. Epinephrine is a drug that is emitted from the adrenal medulla, passing across the bloodstream to the brain to exert its effects on several tissues of the body. The impacts of the catecholamine's on the different tissues of the body are very involved and maybe the subject of a research paper. The primary function of catecholamine metabolites affecting the ketogenic diet was to increase fatty acids excretion in the urine and increase fatty acids in the blood. When it's hard for someone to change their ways, it's because their insulin levels aren't where they should be. The only hormone that actually affects fat mobilization is insulin. Like the Catecholamine's, insulin and insulin mimics have a corresponding effect on fat mobilization.

3. Liver glycogen

The liver is one of the most metabolically active organs in the whole human body. Although everything we consume is not digested immediately by the stomach, this is part of the whole digestion process. Like the body, the degree to which the liver retains glycogen is the dominating influence to the extent to which the body will retain or break down nutrients. It is typically (hesitation) because there is a higher body fat level associated with elevated liver glycogen levels. The liver is analogous to a short term stead storehouse and glycogen source regulating blood glucose in our body. After the liver releases more glucose into the blood, more glucagon is released, which activates the breaking down of liver glycogen to glucose, to be introduced into the bloodstream. When the liver has glycogen stocks completely, blood glucose levels are retained, and the body enters the anabolic state, meaning the incoming glucose, amino acids, and free fatty acids are all processed as these three molecules, respectively. This is often referred to as 'the fed establishment.' Red blood cells can't hold as much oxygen as they did when filled with massive amounts of glycogen, so they release it when they're no longer needed and transform into the liver. The body cuts edible protein into amino acids, which are then placed into the formation of amino acids, and finally, will produce for you fats and sugars. This is often referred to as the 'fasted' condition.

4. Enzyme levels

Precise control of fuel consumption in the body is done through the action of enzymes. Ultimately, enzyme levels are calculated by the carbohydrates that are being consumed in the diet and the hormone levels which are caused by it. On the other hand, where there is a surplus of carbohydrates in one's diet, this form of dietary shift stimulates insulin's influence on the cells' ability to utilize glucose and prevent fatty stores' degradation. Thus, if there is a decrease in insulin levels, the enzymes are blocked, which results in a drop in the enzymes involved in glucose usage and in fats breakdown. A long term adjustment to a high carbohydrate / low carbohydrate diet may induce longer-term modifications in the enzymes involved in fats and carbohydrates, resulting in long term changes in the core. If you limit carbohydrate consumption for many weeks, this will deplete enzymes' liver and muscle and transfer them to be brought upon the liver and muscle that concerns fat burning. The result of disrupting the balance of dietary components is an inability to use carbs for fuel for some time after food is reintroduced to the diet.

Chapter 3: Keto with Intermittent Fasting

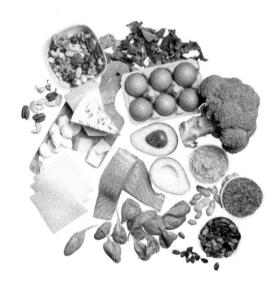

This chapter will give you a detailed view to the Keto with intermittent fasting.

Intermittent fasting, in a more condensed definition, allows people to miss a meal daily. The popular forms of intermittent fasting include the one day fast, a 24 hour fast or a 5:2 fast, where people eat very little food for a predetermined number of days, then consume lots of food (ADF). The intermittent fasting function of IF breaks the subjects fasting routine every other day. Unlike crash diets that frequently produce rapid results but can be hard to sustain for the long run, both intermittent fasting and keto Diet focus on the real root systems of how the body absorbs food and how you make your dietary decisions for each day. Intermittent eating and Keto diets should be practiced as dietary modification. They are long-term options for a better, happier you.

It is where the biggest distinction lies among IF and Interval feeding (TRF). The TRF is the fast of restricting the feeding time to between 4-10 hours during the day and missing the fasting time the rest of the time. All or most people who observe intermittent fasting do so regularly.

3.1. What Is Ketosis?

From the outside looking in, carbs appear to be a simple and fast means of bringing nutrients right through the day. Think of all those grab-and-go and protein-filled snacks that we equate with breakfast—granola bars, fruit-filled muffins, smoothies. We start our mornings by eating many carbs, and then later on in the day, they add more carbs. Just because a given technology works does not make it the most effective way. To keep us safe, the tissues and cells that produce our bodies require energy to fulfil their daily functions. There are two main sources of strength in the foods we consume, but the first source is non-animal, and the second source is animal. One source of energy is the carbohydrate, which transforms into glucose. At this time, this is the process that most people go through. These cars have an alternative fuel, however, and a shocking one: fat. No, the very thing any doctor has recommended you to reduce your lifelong lifespan may be the weapon you need to jump-start your metabolism. During this process, tiny organic molecules, called Ketone, are emitted from our body, signalling that the food we eat is being broken down. Ketones are actual nutrients that help run much of our body's cells, including muscles. You've undoubtedly heard the term "Metabolism" repeated in one's life, but do you understand what it means exactly as a fast-acting chemical process? In short, this is alkaline, causing effective cellular functioning, which can be present in any type of living thing. Considering that humans are extremely difficult in many ways, our bodies generally process simpler things like food and exercise. Our bodies are actively struggling to do their jobs. And whether we are either asleep or not, our cells are actively constructing and restoring. The robots ought to remove the energetic particles from inside our bodies.

Around the same time, glucose, which is what carbohydrates are broken down into after we ingest them, is a critical component in the process of bringing sugar into the body. We are now concentrating our diet on carbs as the main source of calories for our body. Without mentioning the fructose we eat as well as the recommended daily servings of fruit, starchy veggies, and starchy vegetables, as well as plant-based sources of protein, there is no shortage of glucose in our bodies. The problem with this type of energy use is that this results in us buying into the recycling-focused consumerism that is a by-product of the half-baked technologies. Our bodies get hammered by the number of calories we eat every day. Some people are eating more than they need, and that can contribute to obesity.

Most people cannot reach ketosis quickly, but you can reach it by exercising, eating less, and drinking a decent amount of water. As was seen through the data, our current "Food Pyramid," which instructs us to consume a high amount of carbohydrate-rich foods as energy sources, is turned upside down. A more effective formula for feeding your body has fats at the top, making up 60 to 80 percent of your diet; protein in the middle at 20 to 30 percent; and carbs (real glucose in disguise) way at the bottom, accounting for only 5 to 10 percent of your regular eating plan.

3.2. Paleo vs. Keto

Evolution has many opportunities to bring. We can use fire and energy to cook our food is evidence enough that change can be a positive thing about our lives. Anywhere between our trapper foraging lifestyle and the industrialized lifestyle we have today, there is a significant disconnect. Although our lifespans have improved, we're not winning from the longevity of those additional years because our health is being undermined. The tired, unclear sensation you are having might be not just because you need to get more sleep - it may be because you lack vitamin B12 in your diet. If we eat food as fuel for our bodies, it's fair to assume that what we eat has a big effect on our productivity. If you burn fuel in an engine designed to run on gasoline, there could be some very harmful consequences. Is it conceivable that our bodies have set up this insulin receptor cascade to only accept sugar, in a process comparable to our transition to providing fat as a rapid source of energy rather than a source of energy for our early ancestors? I know this sounds an awful lot like arguing for a Paleo diet, but although the ketogenic lifestyle seems similar, keto's basic concept is vastly different. Ketosis happens when you eat fewer calories and change the intake of protein and fat. There are many medicinal effects of ketosis, and the primary one is quick weight loss (fat, protein, carbohydrates, fiber, and fluids). Per calorie is made up of four distinct types of macronutrients. Many considerations go into the certain food decisions that a person makes, and it's crucial to consider one's emotions.

Fiber makes us regular, for instance, and it lets food flows into the digestive tract. What goes in has to come out, and for that process, fiber is necessary. Protein helps to heal tissue, generate enzymes and to create bones, muscles and skin. Liquids keep us hydrated; our cells, muscles, and organs do not operate correctly without them. The primary function of carbohydrates is to supply energy, but the body must turn them into glucose to do so, which has a ripple effect on the body's parts. Because of its link to insulin production through higher blood sugar levels, a carb intake is a balancing act for persons with diabetes. Good fats stimulate cell formation, protect our lungs, help keep us warm, and supply nutrition, but only in small amounts when carbs are ingested. I'm going to explain more about when and how this is happening soon.

3.3. Carbs vs. Net Carbs

In virtually any food supply, carbohydrates occur in some type. Total carbohydrate reduction is unlikely and unrealistic. To work, we want some carbohydrates. If we want to learn that certain foods that drop into the restricted group on a keto diet become better options than others, it's important to understand this.

In the caloric breakdown of a meal, fiber counts as a carb. It is interesting to remember is that our blood sugar is not greatly impaired by fiber, a positive thing because it is an integral macronutrient that allows us better digest food. You're left with what's considered net carbs after subtracting the sum of fiber from the number of carbs in the caloric tally of an element or finished recipe. Think of your pay check before (gross) taxes and after (net). A bad comparison, maybe, because no one wants to pay taxes, but an efficient one to try to explain and track carbs versus net carbs. You place a certain amount of carbohydrates in your bloodstream, but any of them does not influence your blood sugar content.

It doesn't mean that with whole-grain pasta, you may go mad. Although it's a better alternative than flour of white-coloured pasta, you can limit your net carbs to 20 - 30 grams per day total. To place that in context, approximately 35 g of carbohydrates and just 7 grams of total fiber are found in two ounces of undercooked whole-grain pasta. Pasta and bread are undoubtedly the two key things people would ask you if you miss them.

3.4. When does ketosis kick in?

Most individuals go through ketosis within a few days. People who are different will take a week to adapt. Factors that cause ketosis include existing body mass, diet, and exercise levels. Ketosis is a moderate state of ketosis since ketone levels would be low for a longer time. One can calculate ketone levels in a structured way, but you can note certain biological reactions that indicate you are in ketosis. There are not as serious or drastic symptoms, and benefits can outweigh risks in this phase-in time, so it is good to be familiar with symptoms in case they arise.

Starvation vs. Fasting

Make a deliberate decision to fast. The biggest differentiator between going on a fast and feeding intermittently is that it is your choice to continue fasting. The amount of time you want to fast and the reason for fasting are not imposed upon you by the hospital, whether it is for religious practices, weight loss, or a prolonged detox cycle. Most fasting is performed at will. When fasting, proper feeding has clear implications on the overall way of our well-being. A series of situations can bring about starvation out of the hands of the people suffering from those conditions. Starvation, hunger, and war are but a couple of these conditions to be caused by a devastated economy. Starvation is starvation due to lack of the proper nutrients that can lead to organ failure and ultimately death. No one wants to live without calories.

When I knew that avoiding smoking would help my health, I immediately wondered, "Why do I continue to smoke?" And once I learn about the motivations for doing this, it is much easier to see them. I have also been concerned about the early days of fasting. Before I knew that there is a distinction between fasting and starvation and that it is safe, my first response to the thought of not eating and starving was still, "Why would anyone choose to kill themselves with starving?." As for this article's intent, someone who fasts is just opting not to eat for a predetermined amount of time. Even nonviolent vigils that are meant to oppose using a certain form of killing feed larger and larger gatherings.

Would your hunger vanish before the fast?

So that's a brilliant query; let's try a couple more angles. The fact is, we all eat a full meal once a day. It is a normal tradition that we eat our last meal a few hours before going to sleep, and all but breastfeeding new-borns do not eat the moment they wake up. And if you devote just a limit of six hours a night to sleep, you are likely to be fasting ten hours a day anyway. Now, let's begin to incorporate the concept in periodic to the formula. Anything that is "intermittent" implies something that is not constant. When adding it to the concept of fasting, it means you're lengthening the time that you don't eat between meals (the term "breakfast" means only that, breaking the fast).

From fasting once a day, we have an established "mind over matter" power. What will be a major concern, though, would be mind over mind. We will come back to the issue of how you feel after you stop feeding. The first week of fasting may change as you get used to the prolonged amount of time of your current intermittent fasting target. All of the fasting periods that I have given allow you time-wise to adapt to the Ketogenic Diet and this method adjusts your sleeping routine so that it suits them. It is conceivable (and likely) that your body will start to feel hungry about 10 a.m., around the moment it usually eats lunch. But, after one day, you can adapt, and after a couple of days, you should no longer have trouble feeding before noon.

To support you before making the shift you're playing with, observe what happens when you put back the first meal of the day by an extra thirty minutes per day for a week. This way, as you begin the schedule set out here, you'll need to change the timing of your final meal of the day just after you begin week two of the plan for the Meals from Noon to 6 p.m. No appointments are required.

3.5. Why Prefer Intermittent Fasting?

Now that you have learned that it is possible to fast without starving to death and that it is also a deliberate decision, you might think, why on earth you would ever choose to fast. Its ability to encourage weight loss is one of the key reasons that IF has taken the diet world by storm. Metabolism is one feature of the human body. Metabolism requires two basic reactions: catabolism and anabolism.

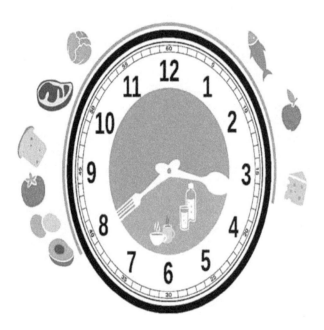

Catabolism is the portion of metabolism where our bodies break down food. Catabolism involves breaking down large compounds into smaller units. The body uses the energy from the food we consume to produce new cells, build muscles, and sustain organs. This term is often referred to as parallel or dual catabolism and anabolism. A diet routine that sees us eating most of the day means our bodies have less time to waste in the anabolic process of metabolism. It is hard to find out since they are related, but note that they occur at different rates. The most significant point is that a prolonged fasting time allows for optimum metabolic efficiency.

The improved mental acuity has an intrinsic influence of improving attention, focus, concentration and focus. According to various reports, fasting made you more alert and concentrated, not sleepy or light-headed. Many people point to nature and our desire to survive. We may not have had food preservation, but we lived day to day, regardless of how ample food supplies may have been.

Scientists agree that fasting often heightens neurogenesis, the growth and regeneration of nerve tissue in the brain. Both paths lead to the fact that fasting gives the body enough time to do routine maintenance. You extend the time you give your body to concentrate on cellular growth and tissue recovery by sleeping longer between your last meal and your first meal.

Are Fluids Allowed While Fasting?

The last important detail for intermittent fasting is that it speeds up the metabolism; unlike religious fasting, which also forbids food consumption during the fast period, an IF requires you to drink a certain liquid during the fast time. You are not consuming something that is caloric; therefore, this action breaks the fast. As we can glean from its strong weight loss record, a closer look through the prism of intermittent fasting can yield very promising outcomes. Bone broth (here) is the beneficiary of both the nutrients and vitamins and can refill the sodium amounts. Permission has been given to use coffee and tea without any sweeteners and ideally without any milk or cream. There are two separate schools of thinking about applying milk or soda to your coffee or tea. Provided it's just a high-fat addition, such as coconut oil or butter to make bulletproof coffee (here), many keto supporters believe it's a waste of time and not properly gain sufficient protein. Using MCT oil, it is assumed that people can obtain more energy and be happier moving on with their daily lives. Coffee and tea drinkers tend toward simple brews. It is perfect for you to choose whichever strategy you want, as long as you don't end up "alternating" between the two techniques. I often recommend drinking water, as staying hydrated is necessary for any healthier choice a person can make. Caffeine use can be very depleting, so be careful to control your water intake and keep yourself balanced.

3.6. The Power of Keto Combined & Intermittent Fasting

When you're in ketosis, the process breaks down fatty acids to create ketones for fuel is basically what the body does to keep things going when you're fasting. Fasting for a few days has a noticeable impact on a carb-based diet. After the initial step of burning carbohydrates for energy, your body transforms to burning fat for heat. You see where I'm going. If it takes 24 to 48 hrs. For the body to turn to fat for food, imagine the consequences of keto. Maintaining ketosis means your body has been trying to burn fat for fuel. Spending a long time in a fasting state means you burn fat. Intermittent starvation combined with keto results in more weight loss than other traditional diets. Extra fat-burning capabilities are due to the gap in time between the last and first meals. Ketosis is used in bodybuilding because it helps shed fat without losing muscle. It's healthy when it's the right weight, and muscle mass is good for fitness.

How does it work?

It is an incredible lifestyle adjustment to turn to the keto diet. Since it can help you consume less, it's better to ease into this program's fasting part. Despite the diet not being entirely fresh, yet has been around for a long time, people seem to respond rapidly to consuming mostly fat, so their body has been accustomed to burning fat for food, but be patient if either of the above occurs: headaches, exhaustion, light-headedness, dizziness, low blood sugars, nausea. A rise in appetite, cravings for carbohydrates, or weight gain. Often make sure you get certain nutrients: brain well-being, fat-burning, testosterone, and mood. Week 2 of the 4-Week schedule begins intermittent fasting, and it is not continued until the 2nd week. During the phase-in process, you'll want to find out what the meals and hours are about. Before integrating the intermittent-fasting portion of your diet, it is recommended that you stop eating your last meal more than six hours in advance. (6 p.m.) It will help you get into a fasting state and help you stop snacking. When you learn how to better nourish your body, you will learn how to reel in the pesky compulsion to feed, and you will be able to maintain a more controlled relationship with your psychological needs as well. When time goes by, cravings inevitably stop. We sometimes associate the craving for food with hunger, when actually the craving for food is due to a learned habit and hunger is a biochemical cue to refuel the body's energy stores.

3.7. Calories vs. Macronutrients

The focus on keto is on tracking the amount of fat, protein, and carbohydrates you eat. It's just a closer examination of every calorie ingested. To decide how many calories you can consume for weight management and weight loss, it is also important to have a baseline metabolic rate called BMR (another reason defining your goals is important). In both your general well-being and achieving and remaining in ketosis, all these macronutrients play a crucial function, but carbohydrates are the one that receives the most attention on keto since they result in glucose during digestion, which is the energy source you are attempting to guide your body away from utilizing. Any study indicates that the actual number of total carbs that one can eat a day on keto is 50 grams or less, resulting in 20 to 35 net carbs a day depending on the fiber content. The lower the net carbohydrates you can get down, the sooner your body goes into ketosis, and the better it's going to be to keep in it.

Bearing in mind that we target around 20 grams of net carbs a day, depending on how many calories you need to eat depending on your BMR, the fat and protein grams are factors. Depending on the exercise level, the recommended daily average for women ranges between 1,600 and 2,000 calories for weight maintenance (from passive to active). According to a daily diet, consuming 160 grams of fat + 70 grams of protein + 20 grams of carbohydrates represents 1,800 calories of intake, the optimal number for weight control for moderately active women in the USDA (walking 1.5 to 3 miles a day). You would like to reach for 130 grams of fat + 60 grams of protein + 20 grams of carbohydrates to jump-start weight loss if you have a sedentary lifestyle, described as having exercise from normal daily activities such as cleaning and walking short distances only (1500 calories).

3.8. The Physical Side Effects of Keto:

Unlike diet programs that merely reduce the weight loss foods you consume, keto goes further. In order to improve how the body turns what you consume into electricity, ketosis is about modifying the way you eat. The ketosis phase changes the equation from burning glucose (remember, carbs) to burning fat for fuel instead. When the body adapts to a different way of working, this comes with potential side effects. This is also why around week two, and not from the get-go, the 4-Week schedule here stages of intermittent fasting. It's important to give yourself time to change properly, both physically and mentally. Keto fever and keto breath are two physical alterations that you may encounter while transitioning to a keto diet.

1. Keto Flu

Often referred to as carb flu, keto flu can last anywhere from a few days to a few weeks. As the body weans itself from burning glucose for energy, metabolic changes occurring inside can result in increased feelings of lethargy, muscle soreness, irritability, light-headedness or brain fog, changes in bowel movements, nausea, stomach aches, and difficulty concentrating and focusing. It sounds bad, I know, and perhaps slightly familiar. Yes, these are all recurrent flu signs, hence the term. The good news is that when your body changes, this is a transient process, and it does not affect everybody. A deficiency of electrolytes (sodium, potassium, magnesium and calcium) and sugar removal from substantially reduced carbohydrate intake are reasons causing these symptoms. Expecting these future effects means that, should anything arise at all, you will be prepared to relieve them and reduce the duration of keto flu.

Sodium levels are specifically affected by the volume of heavily processed foods you eat. To explain, all we eat is a processed food; the word means "a series of steps taken to achieve a specific end." The act of processing food also involves cooking from scratch at home. However, these heavily processed foods appear to produce excessive amounts of secret salt in contrast to our present society, where ready-to-eat foods are available at any turn of the store (sodium is a preservative as well as a flavour modifier).

Other foods to concentrate on during your keto phase-in time are given below. They're a rich supply of minerals such as magnesium, potassium and calcium to keep the electrolytes in check.

- Potassium is important for hydration. It is present in Brussels sprouts, asparagus, salmon, tomatoes, avocados, and leafy greens.
- Seafood, Avocado, Spinach, Fish, and Vegetables that are high in magnesium can greatly assist with Cramps and Muscle Soreness.
- Calcium can promote bone health and aid in the absorption of nutrients.
- Including cheese, nuts, and seeds like almonds, broccoli, bok Choy, sardines, lettuce, sesame and chia seeds.

The other option that people evaluate to prevent the keto flu is to start eating less refined carbohydrates to lessen the chances of experiencing the keto flu. It can be as simple as making a few simple changes in what you eat, replacing the muffin with a hard-boiled or scrambled egg, replacing the bun with lettuce (often referred to as protein-style when ordering), or switching out spaghetti with zoodles. This way, when you dive into the plan here or here, it'll feel more like a gradual step of eating fewer carbohydrates than a sudden right turn in your diet.

2. Keto Breath

Let's dig into the crux of the matter first. Poor breath is basically a stench. But, it's a thing you can prepare yourself for when transitioning to the ketosis diet. There are two related hypotheses there might be a reason for this. When the body reaches ketosis (a state whereby it releases a lot of energy), which makes your fat a by-product of acid, more acetone is released by the body (yes, the same solvent found in nail polish remover and paint thinners). Any acetone is broken down in the bloodstream in a process called decarboxylation in order to get it out of the body into the urine and breathe in the acetone. It can cause that a person has foul-smelling breath.

When protein is also present in the keto breath, it adds a mildly gross sound. You must note that the macronutrient target is a high fat, mild protein, and low carb. People make the mistake that high fat is interchangeable with high protein. It is not a real assertion at all. The body's metabolism between fat and protein varies. Our bodies contain ammonia when breaking down protein, and all of the ammonia is normally released in our urine production. When you eat more protein or more than you should, the excess protein is not broken or digested and goes to your gut. With time, the extra protein will turn to ammonia and releasing by your breath.

3.9. The Fundamentals of Ketogenic Diet

The keto diet regimen involves eating moderately low carb, high sugar, and mild protein to train the body to accept fat as its basic food. Continuing the procedure, I would add a Keto diet to my diet. Since the body may not have carbohydrate stores, it burns through its glycogen supplies rapidly. It is when the body appears to be in a state of emergency since it has run out of food. At this stage, the body goes into ketosis, and this is when you start using fat as the primary source of power. It typically occurs within three days of beginning the drug. Then, the body transforms the fat onto itself, usually taking over three months and a half to complete the transition. You are well accustomed to fat. So if you aren't feeding the body properly, that's why the body takes advantage of your own fat deposits (fasting).

The Keto Diet Advantage for Intermittent Fasting

Before entering intermittent fasting, keto advises four a month and a half to be on the keto diet. You're not going to be better off eating fat alone, so you're going to have less yearning. The keto diet in contemplates was all the more satisfying, and people encountered less yearning. In contrast, keto also showed its bulk storage ability and was best at maintaining digestion.

Sorts of Intermittent Fasting

This technique involves fasting two days a week and on some days actually eating 500 calories. You will have to observe a typical, healthy keto diet for the next five days. Because fasting days are allotted just 500 calories, you will need to spend high-protein and fat nutrients to keep you satisfied. Only made mindful that there is a non-fasting day in the middle of both.

1. Time-Restricted Eating

For the most part, because your fasting window involves the time you are dozing, this fasting approach has proven to be among the most popular. The swift 16/8 means that you are fast for sixteen hours and eat for eight hours. That might believe it is only allowed to eat from early afternoon until 8 p.m. and start quickly until the next day. The incredible thing about this technique is that it doesn't have to be 16/8; at the moment, you can do 14/10 and get equivalent incentives.

2. Interchange Day Fasting

Despite the 5:2 strategy and time restriction, this alternative allows you to be rapid every other day, normally limiting yourself from around 500 calories on fasting. The non-fasting days would actually be consumed normally. It can be an exhausting strategy that can make others hesitate when it is difficult to keep up with it.

3. 24 Hour Fast

I called, for short, "One Meal a Day" or OMAD, otherwise. This speed is sustained for an entire 24 hours and is usually done just a few days a week. Next, you'll need some inspiration to resume fasting to prop you up.

Keeping up the Motivation

It can be hard to stick to an eating and fasting regimen on the off chance that you are short on ideas, so how do you keep it up? The accompanying focus will help to concentrate on your general goals by presenting basic path reasons.

Chapter 4: Top 20 Keto Recipes

In this chapter, we will discuss some delicious keto recipes.

4.1. Muffins of Almond Butter

(Ready in 35 Mins, Serves: 12, Difficulty: Normal)

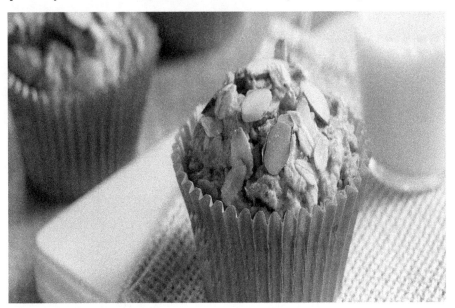

Ingredients:

- Four eggs
- 2 cups almond flour
- 1/4 tsp. salt
- 3/4 cup warm almond butter,
- 3/4 cup almond milk
- 1 cup powdered erythritol
- Two teaspoons baking powder

Instructions:

1. In a muffin cup, put the paper liners before the oven is preheated to 160 degrees Celsius.

2. Mix erythritol, almond meal, baking powder, and salt in a mixing bowl.

3. In another cup, mix the warm almond milk with the almond butter.

4. Drop some ingredients in a dry bowl till they are all combined.

5. In a ready cooker, sprinkle the flour and cook for 22-25 minutes until a clean knife is placed in the center.

6. Cool the bottle for five minutes to cool.

4.2. Breakfast Quesadilla

(Ready in 25 Mins, Serves: 4, Difficulty: Easy)

Ingredients:

- 4 eggs
- 1/4 cup (56 g) salsa
- 1/4 cup (30 g) low-fat Cheddar cheese, shredded
- 8 corn tortillas

Instructions:

1. When it is done, throw in the salsa, and whisk in the cheese to the very top. Sprinkle the oil on a few tortillas and then place a few pieces on an even number of the tortillas' edges.

2. Take the baking sheet. Divide the egg mixture between the tortillas, which is much more challenging. Oil-side up, cover the remaining tortillas. For 3 minutes or before the golden brown heats up, grill the quesadillas on each side. Serve.

4.3. California Breakfast Sandwich

(Ready in 30 Mins, Serves: 6, Difficulty: Easy)

Ingredients:

- 1/2 a cup (90 g) chopped tomato
- 1/2 a cup (60 g) grated Cheddar cheese
- Six whole-wheat English muffins
- 2 ounces (55 g) mushrooms, sliced
- One avocado, sliced
- 6 eggs
- 3/4 cup (120 g) chopped onion
- 1 tbsp. unsalted butter

Instructions:

Beat the eggs together. Brown onion in a large oven-proof or high-sided skillet until clear. It's safe and tidy. Chop up avocado, tomatoes, and champagne onion blend and stir. Blend together. Proofread the attached work. Quickly cook until it's almost cooked. Add the salt, vinegar, and cheese. Spoon with English toasted muffins.

4.4. Stromboli Keto

(Ready in 45 Mins, Serves: 4, Difficulty: Normal)

Ingredients:

- 4 oz. ham
- 4 oz. cheddar cheese
- Salt and pepper
- 4 tbsp. almond flour

- 1¼ cup shredded mozzarella cheese

- 1 tsp. Italian seasoning

- 3 tbsp. coconut flour

- One egg

Instructions:

1. To avoid smoking, stir the mozzarella cheese in the microwave for 1 minute or so.

2. Apply each cup of the melted mozzarella cheese, mix the food, coconut fleece, pepper and salt together. A balanced equilibrium. Then add the eggs and blend again for a while after cooling off.

3. Place the mixture on the parchment pad and place the second layer above it. Through your hands or rolling pin, flatten it into a rectangle.

4. Remove the top sheet of paper and use a butter knife to draw diagonal lines towards the dough's middle. They can be cut one-half of the way on the one side. And cut diagonal points on the other side, too.

5. At the edge of the dough are alternate ham and cheese slices. Then fold on one side, and on the other side, cover the filling.

6. Bake for 15-20 minutes at 226°C; place it on a baking tray.

4.5. Cups of Meat-Lover Pizza

(Ready in 26 Mins, Serves: 12, Difficulty: Easy)

Ingredients:

- 24 pepperoni slices

- 1 cup cooked and crumbled bacon

- 12 tbsp. sugar-free pizza sauce

- 3 cups grated mozzarella cheese

- 12 deli ham slices

- 1 lb. bulk Italian sausage

Instructions

1. Preheat the oven to 375 F Celsius (190 degrees Celsius). Italian brown sausages, soaked in a saucepan of extra fat.

2. Cover the 12-cup ham slices with a muffin tin. Divide it into sausage cups, mozzarella cheese, pizza sauce, and pepperoni slots.

3. Bake for 10 mins at 375. Cook for 1 minute until the cheese pops and the meat tops show on the ends, until juicy.

4. Enjoy the muffin and put the pizza cups to avoid wetting them on paper towels. Uncover or cool down and heat up quickly in the toaster oven or microwave.

4.6. Chicken Keto Sandwich

(Ready in 30 Mins, Serves: 2, Difficulty: Normal)

Ingredients:

For the Bread:

- 3 oz. cream cheese
- ⅛ tsp. cream of tartar Salt
- Garlic powder
- Three eggs

For the Filling:

- 1 tbsp. mayonnaise
- Two slices bacon
- 3 oz. chicken
- 1 tsp. Sriracha
- 2 slices pepper jack cheese
- 2 grape tomatoes
- ¼ avocado

Instructions:

1. Divide the eggs into several cups. Add cream tartar, cinnamon, then beat to steep peaks in the egg whites.

2. In a different bowl, beat the cream cheese. In a white egg mixture, combine the mixture carefully.

3. Place the batter on paper and, like bread pieces, make little square shapes. Gloss over the garlic powder, then bake for 25 mins at 148°C.

4. As the bread bakes, cook the chicken and bacon in a saucepan and season to taste.

5. Remove from the oven and cool when the bread is finished for 10-15 mins. Then add mayo, Sriracha, tomatoes, and mashed avocado, and add fried chicken and bacon to your sandwich.

4.7. Keto Tuna Bites With Avocado

(Ready in 13 Mins, Serves: 8, Difficulty: Very Easy)

Ingredients:

- 10 oz. drained canned tuna
- ⅓ cup almond flour
- ½ cup coconut oil
- ¼ cup mayo
- 1 avocado
- ½ tsp. garlic powder
- ¼ tsp. onion powder
- ¼ cup parmesan cheese
- Salt and pepper

Instructions:

1. Both ingredients are mixed in a dish (excluding cocoa oil). Shape small balls of almond meal and fill them.

2. Fry them with coconut oil (it needs to be hot) in a medium-hot pan until browned on all sides.

4.8. Green Keto Salad

(Ready in 10 Mins, Serves: 1, Difficulty: Easy)

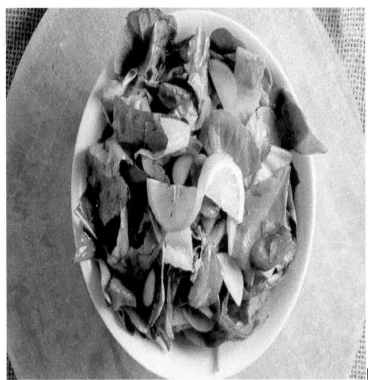

Ingredients:

- 100 g mixed lettuce
- 200 g cucumber
- 2 stalks celery
- 1 tbsp. olive oil
- Salt as per choice
- 1 tsp white wine vinegar or lemon juice

Instructions:

1. With your hands, rinse and cut the lettuce.

2. Cucumber and celery chop.

3. Combine all.

4. For the dressing, add vinegar, salt, and oil.

4.9. Breakfast Enchiladas

(Ready in 1 Hr., Serves: 8, Difficulty: Normal)

Ingredients:

- 12 ounces (340 g) ham, finely chopped
- Eight whole-wheat tortillas
- 4 eggs
- 1 tbsp. flour
- 1/4 tsp. garlic powder
- 1 tsp. Tabasco sauce
- 2 cups (300 g) chopped green bell pepper
- 1 cup (160 g) chopped onion
- 2 1/2 a cup (300 g) grated Cheddar cheese
- 2 cups (475 ml) skim milk
- 1/2 a cup (50 g) chopped scallions

Instructions:

1. Preheat the oven to 350 °F (180 °C). Combine the ham, scallions, bell pepper, tomatoes and cheese. Apply five teaspoons of the mixture to each tortilla and roll-up.

2. In a 30 x 18 x 5-cm (12 x 7 x 2-inch) non-stick pan. In a separate oven, beat together the eggs, milk, garlic, and Tabasco. Cook for 30 minutes with foil, then show the last 10 minutes.

Tip: Serve with a sour cream dollop, salsa, and slices of avocado.

4.10. Keto Mixed Berry Smoothie Recipe

(Ready in 5 Mins, Serves: 4, Difficulty: Easy)

Ingredients:

- 2 scoops Vanilla Collagen
- 1 cup of frozen Mixed Berries
- 2 cups Ice
- 1/4 cup Erythritol Powdered Monk Fruit
- 1 cup Unsweetened Coconut Milk Vanilla

Instructions

1. In a high-speed blender, combine all the ingredients.

2. Use or mix until smooth the "smoothie" setting.

4.11. Low-Carb Tropical Pink Smoothie

(Ready in 5 Mins, Serves: 1, Difficulty: Easy)

Ingredients: (makes 1 smoothie)

- $^1/_2$ small dragon fruit
- 1 tbsp. chia seeds
- 1 small wedge Gallia, Honeydew
- 1/2 a cup coconut milk *or* heavy whipping cream
- 1 scoop of whey protein powder (vanilla or plain), or gelatin or egg white powder.
- 3-6 drops extract of Stevia *or* other low-carb sweeteners
- 1/2 a cup water
- *Optional:* few ice cubes

Instructions

1. Monitor and place all the components smoothly in a mixer and pulse. Before or after combining this, you can apply the ice.

2. It is possible to include the fruit of a white or pink dragon. Serve.

4.12. Keto Peanut Butter Smoothie

(Ready in 1 Min, Serves: 1, Difficulty: Very Easy)

Ingredients:

- 1/2 a cup almond milk
- 1 tbsp. peanut butter

- 1 tbsp. cocoa powder
- 1-2 tbsp. peanut butter powdered
- 1/4 of avocado
- 1 serving liquid stevia
- 1/4 cup ice

Instructions

1. Add all the ingredients other than the ice and mix well in a food processor.

2. Apply enough milk to the smoothie for the ideal consistency. Add more ice or ground peanut butter to thin it out.

3. Serve it in a glass.

4.13. 5 Minute Keto Cookies & Cream Milkshake

(Ready in 5 Mins, Serves: 2, Difficulty: Easy)

Ingredients:

- $3/4$ cup heavy whipping cream or coconut milk
- Two large squares of grated dark chocolate
- **Optional:** frozen cubes of almond milk/ few ice cubes
- 1 cup unsweetened any nut or almond milk or seed milk
- 1 tsp vanilla powder or vanilla extract sugar-free
- 1-2 tsp Erythritol powdered, few drops of stevia
- $1/3$ cup walnuts or pecans chopped
- 2 tbsp. almond butter, (roasted or sunflower seed)
- 2 tbsp. coconut cream /whipped cream for garnishing

Instructions

1. Place in a blender, mix all the ingredients together (except topping). It is thicker as you blink. The ganache should be lit or topped with other ingredients.

2. Mix the whipped cream into the topping separately. Use 1/2 to 1 cup of milk for pounding. You should have whipped cream in the fridge for three days.

3. Pour some water into a bottle. Drizzle the nuts and butter leftover over the milk.

4.14. Keto Eggnog Smoothie

(Ready in 5 Mins, Serves: 1, Difficulty: Easy)

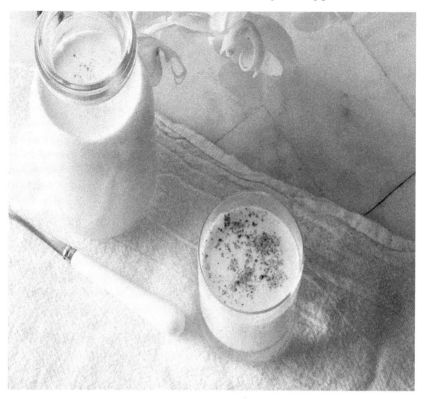

Ingredients:

- 1 Large Egg
- 1 tsp Erythritol
- 1/4 cup whipping cream (coconut cream for dairy-free)
- 1/2 tsp Cinnamon
- 4 Cloves ground approx. ¼ tsp
- 1 tsp Maple Syrup Sugar-Free (optional)

Instructions

In a blender, combine all the ingredients and mix fast for 30 seconds – 1 min.

4.15. Easy Keto Oreo Shake

(Ready in 5 Mins, Serves: 2, Difficulty: Easy)

Ingredients:

- 4 large eggs
- 2 tbsp. black cocoa powder or Dutch-process cocoa powder
- 1 1/2 cups unsweetened cashew milk, almond milk, or water 4 tbsp. roasted almond butter or Keto Butter
- 3 tbsp. Erythritol powdered or Swerve
- 1/4 cup whipping cream
- 1/4 tsp vanilla powder or 1/2 tsp vanilla extract (sugar-free)
- 1/2 a cup whipped cream for garnishing

•

Instructions

1. Place the frozen or cashew milk/almond milk in an ice cube tray and then freeze them. Under the right conditions (which means don't freeze the shake), miss this step and go on to the next.

2. Stir the cream in a tub of frozen milk. To produce ice cream, add ice cream to the warmed cream. Put some ova somewhere.

3. Apply the soaked nuts, sweetener, cacao powder, and vanilla to the dish. With macadamia, cocoa, cassava, and MCT, these oils are nice to use with MCT oil. Blend until smooth.

6. Apply more whipped cream before serving.

4.16. Keto Eggs Florentine

(Ready in 55 Mins, Serves: 4, Difficulty: Normal)

Ingredients:

- 1 tbsp. of white vinegar
- 1 Cup cleaned, the spinach leaves fresh
- 2 Tablespoons of Parmesan cheese, finely grated
- 2 Chickens
- 2 Eggs
- Ocean salt and chili to compare

Instructions:

1. Boil the spinach in a decent bowl or steam until it waves.

2. Sprinkle with the parmesan cheese to taste.

3. Break and put the bits on a tray. Place the tray on them.

4. Steam a hot water bath, add the vinegar and mix it in a whirlpool with a wooden spoon.

5. Place the egg in the center of the egg, turn the heat over and cover until set (3-4 minutes). Repeat for the second seed.

6. Put the spinach with the egg and drink.

4.17. Loaded Cauliflower (Low Carb, Keto)

(Ready in 20 Mins, Serves: 4, Difficulty: Easy)

Ingredients:

- 1 pound cauliflower
- 3 tablespoons butter

- 4 ounces of sour cream
- 1/4 tsp. garlic powder
- 1 cup cheddar cheese, grated
- 2 slices bacon crumbled and cooked
- 2 tbsp. chives snipped
- pepper and salt to taste

Instructions

1. Chop or dice cauliflower and switch to a microwave-safe oven. Add two water teaspoons and cover with sticking film. Microwave for 5-10 minutes until thoroughly cooked and tender. Empty the excess water, give a minute or two to dry. If you want to strain the cooking water, steam up your cooling flora (or use hot water as normal.)

2. Add the cauliflower to the food processor. Pulse it until smooth and creamy. Mix in the sugar, garlic powder and sour cream. Press it in a cup, then scatter with more cheese, then mix it up. Add pepper and salt.

3. Add the leftover cheese, chives and bacon to the loaded cauliflower. Place the cauliflower under the grill for a few minutes in the microwave to melt the cheese.

4. Serve and enjoy.

4.18. Crispy Drumsticks

(Ready in 1 Hr. 5 Mins, Serves: 4, Difficulty: Normal)

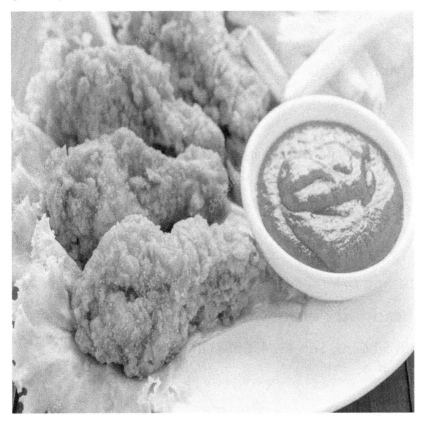

Ingredients:

- Dried thyme
- Olive oil
- 10 – 12 chicken drumsticks (preferably organic)
- Paprika
- Sea salt
- Black pepper

- 4 tbsp. Grass-fed butter or ghee, melted and divided

Instructions

1. Heat the oven to 375 F.

2. Line a rimmed baking sheet.

3. On the parchment paper, in a single sheet of holes between the drumsticks.

4. Mix 1/2 of the melted butter or ghee in olive oil with drumsticks.

5. Sprinkle on thyme and seasoning.

6. Turn it on for 30 minutes. Carefully empty the bottle and switch drumsticks over. When the drumsticks are cooling, produce a thyme and butter mixture again.

7. Return the pie for another 30 minutes (or until finely browned and externally baked).

4.18. Shredded Herbal Cattle

(Ready in 50 Mins, Serves: 4, Difficulty: Normal)

Ingredients:

- 2 tablespoons of rice wine
- 1 tbsp. of olive oil
- 1 pound leg,
- 2 Chipotle peppers in adobo sauce,
- 1 garlic clove chopped,
- Mature tomatoes, peeled and pureed
- 1 yellow onion
- 1/2 tbsp. chopped fresh Mustard

- 1 cup of dried basil
- 1 cup of dried marjoram
- 1/4 cut into strips beef
- 2 medium shaped chipotles crushed
- 1 cup beef bone broth
- Table salt and ground black pepper,
- Parsley, 2 spoonful's of new chives, finely chopped

Instructions:

In an oven, steam the oil in a medium to high heat. Continuously cook beef for six to seven minutes. Add all the ingredients to the beef. Heat and cook for 40 minutes; add the remaining to a moderate-low heat. Then tear the meat, have it.

4.19. Nilaga Filipino Soup

(Ready in 45 Mins, Serves: 4, Difficulty: Normal)

Ingredients:

- 1 Tsp. butter
- 1 tbsp. patis (fish sauce)
- 1 pound of pork ribs, boneless and 1 shallot thinly sliced bits,
- Split 2 garlic cloves, chopped 1 (1/2) "slice of fresh ginger, 1 cup chopped
- 1 cup of fresh tomatoes,
- 1 cup pureed "Corn."
- Cauliflower

- salt and green chili pepper, to taste

Instructions:

1. Melt the butter in a bowl over medium to high heat. Heat the pork ribs for 5-6 minutes on both sides. Stir in the shallot, the garlic and the ginger. Add extra ingredients.

2. Cook, sealed, for 30 to 35 mins. Serve in different containers and remain together.

4.20. Lemon Mahi-Mahi Garlicky

(Ready in 30 Mins, Serves: 4, Difficulty: Normal)

Ingredients:

- Kosher salt
- 4 (4-oz.) mahi-mahi fillets
- Ground black pepper
- 1 lb. asparagus
- 2 tbsp. extra-virgin olive oil,
- 1 lemon
- juice of 1 lemon and zest also
- 3 cloves garlic
- ¼ tsp. of crushed red pepper flakes
- 3 tbsp. butter, divided
- 1 tbsp. freshly parsley chopped, and more for garnish

Instructions:

1. Melt one tbsp. Cook some butter in a large saucepan, then add oil. Season with salt and black pepper. Mahia, add, sauté. Cook for 5 minutes on each side. Transfer to a dish.

2. Apply one tbsp. of oil for the casserole. Cook for 4 minutes and add the spawn. Season with salt and pepper on a pan.

3. Heat butter to the skillet. Add garlic and pepper flakes and simmer until fragrant. Then add lemon zest, juice, and Persil. Break the mahi-mahi into smaller pieces, then add asparagus and sauce.

4. Garnish before consuming.

Conclusions:

An important element to note is eating a great combination of lean meat, greens, and unprocessed carbs. The most efficient way to eat a balanced diet is simply adhering to whole foods, mainly because it is a healthy solution. It is crucial to understand that it is impossible to complete a ketogenic diet.

If you're a woman over 50, you may be far more interested in weight loss. Many women experience decreased metabolism at this age at a rate of about 50 calories per day. It can be incredibly hard to control weight gain by slowing the metabolism combined with less activity, muscle degradation and the potential for greater cravings. Many food options can help women over 50 lose weight and maintain healthy habits, but the keto diet has recently been one of the most popular.

Keto Diet for Beginners

Beginners

Step-by-step Guide for Women Over 50 with Recipes For Rapid Weight Loss

By Jason Smith

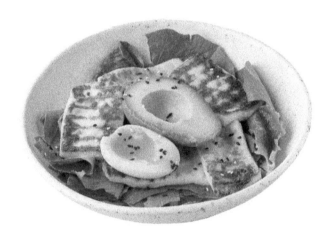

reparation, damages, or monetary loss due to the information herein, either directly or indirectly.

Respective authors own all copyrights not held by the publisher.

The information herein is offered for informational purposes solely and is universal as such. The presentation of the information is without a contract or any type of guarantee assurance.

The trademarks that are used are without any consent, and the publication of the trademark is without permission or backing by the trademark owner. All trademarks and brands within this book are for clarifying purposes only and are owned by the owners themselves, not affiliated with this document.

Introduction

The present accessibility of data implies all that we need to think about anything is readily available, or with one swipe. That same accessibility can often leave you with an excess of knowledge. How would you interpret everything and decide whether intermittent fasting and keto are ideal for you? That is the objective of this book. We did a profound plunge on such lifestyles and analyzed the benefits such practices implemented on their own and combined so you'll cut straight to the chase and acquire started on your intermittent keto venture. Before you set out making changes, approach this as you would any recipe, read the directions from start to end. Ensure you comprehend not exactly how to do intermittent fasting and cook keto-accommodating suppers but the science behind it. Perusing all the starting material will make the progress to this new way of life simpler and help you see the perfect results at the end. Enticing as it is very easy maybe to jump directly to the Meal Plan and recipes. Remember that a strong base is a way to progress. The words between this presentation and the plans give the blocks and mortar to assemble a strong beginning.

It drives us to a decision to vigorously alter our physical body weight or figure because we are not satisfied with our normal body shape or height. Any effort in the name of weight loss is referred to as dieting. A study said that Americans normally invest more than $40 billion a year on dieting and diet-related items. It is often recorded that at some point in time or typically after the age of 50, 60% of women are trying to lose weight. There are too many common methods of dieting or shaping the form or size of the body of which the method of a ketogenic diet (in the short-term, keto) is so well established. A ketogenic diet is a meal with an appropriate protein intake, low in carbohydrates, and heavy in fat consumption. Typically, `ketogenic diet is viewed as a daunting regimen to adopt. It becomes a convenient routine, however, with practice and an understanding of what the diet targets are to attain. The underlying goal is to shift the main fuel supply of the body from carbohydrates such as sugar and bread to fats. It can be done by increasing the consumption of fats and significantly reducing the intake of carbohydrates. The actual effort is that the meal portion is so restrictive like all foodstuffs eaten must be weighed out to a 10th of a gram in meal preparations, and the one who diets may not eat anything which is not "recommended" by the dietician. The level of carbohydrates permitted is very small so that even the minor quantity of sugar in most liquid or chewable pills will avert the diet from working.

Chapter 1: Introduction to Ketogenic Diet

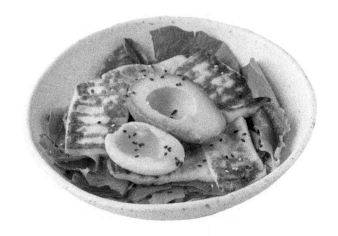

Before conversing the particulars of a ketogenic diet, it is useful to discuss some preliminary information. This contains a general overview of a ketogenic diet procedure as well as the history of its growth, equally for medical situations as well as for fat loss. Intermittent fasting and ketosis, (Known as IF and Keto) target the core system of how you consume food or the selections you make with every meal. Fulfilled properly, keto is life changes, and lasting solutions for a healthy, happy, and smart you.

Carbohydrates on the surface, are a rapid, often fast, and inexpensive form of nutrition to get power throughout the day. Recall all those grab-and-go snacks we associate with our breakfast. Those granola bars, smoothies with fruit-filled, muffins. We resume our mornings with carbs, and as the day progresses, we keep piling them on. Only because anything works doesn't mean that it's the right way to do it. To keep us alive, the tissues and cells that make up our bodies require energy to perform daily functions. There are two main sources from which the foods we consume will derive nutrition. Carbohydrates, which transform into glucose, are one source of nutrition. It is the latest current model that is adopted by most of us. However, there is an alternate fuel, and an interesting one: fat. Yeah, the very thing that you've been advised to restrict your whole life might just be the niche you need to improve your metabolism. When our bodies metabolize food and break down fatty acids, organic compounds, called ketones, are released. To keep our cells and muscles functioning, ketones serve as electricity. Throughout your life, you have undoubtedly used the word "metabolism," but do you know exactly what it means? The word refers to the chemical reactions needed to remain alive in any living organism. Of course, considering the intricacies of the human body, our metabolism is anything but simply gives the complexities to the human body. Our bodies are at work endlessly, even when we sleep, our cells actively construct and rebuild themselves. They need to be able to draw energy from our bodies. One way to fuel our metabolism is glucose, which is what carbohydrates are broken down into after we consume them. As the main energy source, our new dietary recommendations concentrate on carbohydrates. Factor in the additional sugar that we consume and the recommended regular portions of berries, starchy vegetables, grains, and protein sources dependent on plants (e.g., beans), and our bodies do not lack glucose. The concern with this energy use paradigm is that it leaves us on one of those wheels spinning like hamsters. We burn energy but get nowhere, especially if we eat more carbohydrates than our bodies can use in a day's work. But that's the other source of energy that I've mentioned: fat. How specifically does it work? Is it feasible to utilize this alternate type of fuel to enable our body to burn energy more effectively, for greater overall health benefits? We're back to the old notion of what you eat is what you are. Except now think about the principal theory instead of as you burn what you eat. It is when it falls into action for ketosis. Switching to a low-carb, high-fat, moderate-protein diet helps the body to reach a state of ketosis, in which you metabolize fat, allowing ketones to be emitted to power the functions of our intricate inner workings. Through the liver when fatty acids are broken down, it produces ketones. It is about equilibrium to maintain a state of ketosis, but not the sort you are accustomed to when it comes to eating. Our present food pyramid, which instructs us to eat an enormous quantity of foods abundant in carbohydrates for energy, turns out to be upside down. Fats at the top make up 60 to 80 percent of your diet; protein in the center at 20 to 30 percent; and carbs (actual glucose in disguise) at the bottom, making for just 5 to 10 percent of your everyday eating schedule. A more effective plan for feeding your body.

1.1. Origin of Ketogenic Diet

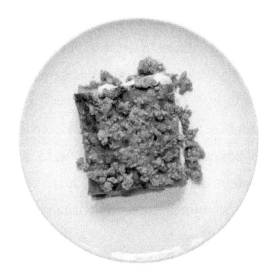

In the first place, we need to discuss the brief history of a ketogenic diet from where it came. a ketogenic diet is not at all a new treatment. In all over history it has been acknowledged that if a person with epilepsy stops eating or fasts, their seizures usually stop. In the earlier time, numerous nutritional "treatments" for epilepsy were introduced, and such cures included the increase or restraint of almost every ingredient such as vegetables, animals, and minerals. Though, fasting or starving as a cure for seizures or attacks was less recognized. Fasting is the only calming measure against epilepsy documented in some researches. Research in the 5th century BC, conducted on a person who had been seized by epileptic fits after having smeared himself before the fire in a bath. Completely abstinence from diet and drink was suggested, and the cure was effective. In the early 20th century, the medicinal use of a ketogenic diet appeared as a tactic to mimic the biochemical effects of fasting. In starting of the 20th century, some physicians present the first scientific research on the importance of fasting in epilepsy. They said the attacks were less during treatment.

Now, let's take a look at history in detail. In the past, several epilepsy nutritional "cures" have been advocated, and those therapies have involved the surplus or limitation of every ingredient (animals, minerals, or vegetables). Additionally, while fasting has been accepted for more than two and a half thousand years as a cure for many illnesses, fasting is less recognized as a remedy for seizures. The only preventive intervention against epilepsy registered in the Hippocratic collection is fasting. Five centuries later, fasting was recorded in Biblical times as a treatment for epilepsy. Mark tells the story of the Jesus treating an epileptic child in a quote from the King James Translation of the Bible (Huisjen, 2000).

In 1911, a pair of Parisian doctors, Gulep and Marie, reported the first modern use of starvation as a cure for epilepsy. They treated 20 children and adults with epilepsy and confirmed that aftercare, seizures became less frequent, although no clear specifics were provided. Contemporary fasting reports from the United States were often reported at the beginning of the 20th century: the first was a study on an osteopathic doctor's patient of Battle Creek's

Dr. Hugh W. Conklin, Michigan; and the second involved Bernarr Macfadden (Freeman et al., 1994). Macfadden was a physical exercise guru/cultist in the early part of the 20th century and a publishing master. He instructed readers about how to physically improve themselves, how to preserve their wellbeing, and how to live with the disease. Every issue of his journal, Physical Culture, held articles about sickly men and women who, by proper diet and exercise, became fit, strong, and attractive. The magazine's distribution had surpassed 500,000 by the close of World War I. Macfadden believed that fasting could relieve and heal just about any condition, including epilepsy, for 3 days to 3 weeks. He had been nationally known, and as part of a plan to be named as the first Health Secretary in 1931, he sought to ingratiate himself with a presidential contender, Franklin D. Roosevelt (Wilkinson, 1997). Dr. Conklin started as Macfadden's assistant and implemented his fasting approach to cure multiple illnesses. It was the fasting procedure of Dr. Conklin to cure epilepsy and the consequences that attracted the interest of another leader in epilepsy science, H. Rawle Geyelin, a New York-Presbyterian Hospital endocrinologist. Dr. Geyelin first recorded his knowledge of fasting as a cure for epilepsy at the American Medical Association Conference in 1921. The leader who records the cognitive development that could arise with fasting was Dr. Geyelin. Dr. Geyelin's lecture was witnessed by Drs. W.G. and Stanley Cobb. Harvard's Lennox. The popularity of Dr. Conklin's fasting outcomes spread steadily and by 1941 it had acquired attention from the Montreal Neurologic Institute in the textbook of Penfield and Erickson on epilepsy. Drs. in the starting of the 1920s, at Harvard Medical School, Cobb and Lennox started researching the impact of hunger on epilepsy therapy. They became the first to notice that there was usually an increase in seizures after 2-3 days. Lennox reported that seizure regulation happened by a transition in the metabolism of the body and that the mere lack of food or starch deprivation in the body caused the body to burn acid-forming fat. Two decisive discoveries were made in 1921. Woodyatt observed that acetone and beta-hydroxybutyric acid occur from malnutrition or a diet comprising too low a carbohydrate proportion and too high a fat proportion in a typical topic (Woodyatt, 1921). At the same time, Dr. Wilder at Mayo Clinic indicated that if ketonemia was created through some methods, the effects of fasting might be achieved (Wilder, 1921). In a sequence of patients with epilepsy, wilder suggested that a ketogenic diet (KD) be attempted. The diet could be as productive as fasting and could be sustained for a much longer period, he suggested. Wilder later published at Mayo Clinic on patients treated with the ketone-producing diet and invented the word "ketogenic diet. In 1925, Peterman at the Clinic named Mayo, eventually reported the KD formula identical to that used today: 1 g of protein per kilogram of body weight in infants, 10-15 g of carbohydrates per day, and the rest of the calories in fat. The value of training caregiver's diet management before discharge, diet individualization, and near follow-up was reported by Peterman. Also, Peterman observed shifts in behavior and cognitive symptoms that followed the KD. These initial findings were soon accompanied by reports from Harvard and McQuarrie and Keith at Mayo Clinic from Talbot et al. In nearly every detailed textbook about epilepsy in kids that came in 1941 and in1980, the use of KD was documented. Most of the material in the book included complete chapters explaining the diet, how to start it, or the ways to measure meal plans. The KD was frequently used in the 1920s, also in the 1930s. In 1972 Livingston, at Johns Hopkins Hospital, published in his textbook on the outcomes of the diet of over 1,000 epilepsy children he had followed in previous decades (Livingston, 1972). He indicated that 52% had absolute regulation of the seizures and a further 27% had increased control.

In the year 1938, diphenylhydantoin was identified by Putnam & Merritt, the interest of researchers moved from the KD's action mode and usefulness to experimental antiepileptic medications. The modern age of epilepsy drug therapy has started and the KD has faded away. In an attempt to render the classic KD more palatable, the medium-chain triglyceride oil diet was developed by Dr. Peter Huttenlocher at the University of Chicago in 1971, enabling some foods to be less limited. The KD was used less and lesser as new antiepileptic medications were available. It was anticipated that this branched fatty acid chain would treat kids formerly put on the regime to treat Lennox-Gastaut syndrome seizures after the advent of sodium valproate and the regimen could no longer be explained. Pediatric neurologists were encouraged to conclude that the rationally designed antiepileptic drugs were the anticipation for the future. Few infants were put on KD, which culminated in fewer dietitians being qualified to use the diet. A scarcity of adequately qualified dietitians means that, without accurate measurement, the KD was frequently applied, contributing to the impression that the diet was unsuccessful. The usage of KD was often based on the understanding of the public. From 1970 to 2000, the usage of KD declined dramatically and PubMed listed just two to eight publications a year. However, when NBC-Dateline TV's broadcast a documentary on the procedure, this shifted drastically when the KD gained mainstream media coverage. A dramatic increase in PubMed publications totaling over 40 a year since then has corresponded with this. This television show was focused on the real tale of Charlie, a 2-year-old child with intractable generalized epilepsy who applied for treatment at Johns Hopkins Hospital out of desperation. Dr. Freeman and Ms. Millicent Kelly (the same dietitian who collaborated with Dr. Livingston) met him and welcomed him to KD. He soon became seizure-free, and his father founded the Charlie Foundation. Informational videos for parents and educational videos for doctors and dietitians regarding KD are disseminated by this foundation. It also helped finance the initial publishing of The Introduction to a Ketogenic Diet: The Epilepsy Diet Cure (Freeman et al., 1994). In 1997, Charlie's father directed the film "First Do No Harm" featuring Meryl Streep, which appeared on national TV. The Foundation sponsored the first multicenter prospective analysis of the KD's effectiveness (Vining et al., 1998).

In recent years, the KD has undergone a re-emergence and modern clinical trials have validated the therapy as being substantially successful (Freeman et al., 1998). KD is currently accessible in over 45 countries around the world (Kossoff &

McGrogan, 2005). However, when this therapy is used by pediatric neurologists, physician perception still has a significant influence. Two recent expert opinion surveys, one conducted in the United States and one conducted in Europe, revealed that KD was the next-to-the-last or last option for almost all childhood epilepsy treatment. Furthermore, a recent study of child neurologists also ranked KD as a therapy that they typically used last, with many not using it at all. There is still a great deal of work to be done to improve the perception of the usefulness of KD, a treatment that compares favorably with other new treatments introduced for the treatment of childhood epilepsy.

Almost a century has passed since the initial use of KD, and many more therapies for children with epilepsy are now available. In the United States, KD has a rich history and continues to be used to treat refractory childhood epilepsy. At almost all major children's hospitals, it is available. Our understanding of the scientific research of this unique therapy has evolved dramatically, resulting in this first international conference dedicated to the KD. A better understanding of the scientific basis of this unique dietary therapy will continue to rise with this renewed scientific interest, resulting in improved epilepsy treatment for all children. This will be an appropriate legacy for the KD.

1.2. Mechanism of Ketosis Diet

A ketogenic diet follows a starving or abstaining state by stopping the body when it requires carbohydrates to function normally, and driving it to metabolize fats. Once the fat is metabolized, ketone bodies are formed. It is the production of the ketone bodies which seems to play a vital role in the accomplishment of a ketogenic diet. When the body starts to produce ketone bodies, it is denoted as the body is in ketosis. It typically takes 3 – 5 days for the body to go into ketosis, once a person starting the diet. Ketosis is easily recognized, because the ketones can be noticed in the urine, and can be recognized by a specific smell of the person's breathing. The prophylactic characteristics of a ketogenic diet form up with time and it may take quite a few weeks before the full outcome of a ketogenic diet is attained.

1.2.1. How does a Ketogenic Diet work?

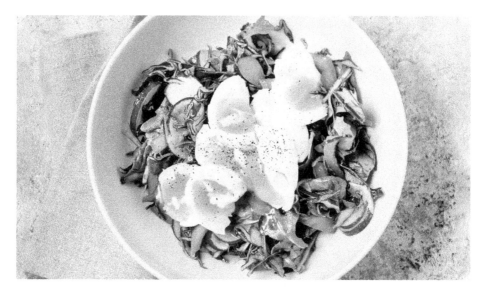

The food we consume provides the fuel which is required to support the body for everyday activity and also provides that material that our body needs to grow. The body is built to use three primary fuels, including carbohydrates, fats, and proteins, unlike vehicles that can only run on oil. Carbohydrates are the primary ingredient of predominantly plant-derived sugars, starch, and wheat.

There are two broad categories of fats: saturated fats, such as butter, mostly derived from livestock, and unsaturated fats, such as corn oil, mostly derived from plants. Protein, finally, comes mostly from plants and is expressed by beef and fish. The above is a large generalization and there are several variants, such as nuts having more than 50% fat. Carbohydrates, fats, and proteins all undergo the same form of chemical reaction, like carbon dioxide and water, for the air we breathe to generate nutrition for the body and waste materials. This is the same response that is noticed when an automobile engine consumes oil or when heat burns wood or coal, etc. While all three fuels in the body are metabolized in the same manner. Carbohydrates, accompanied by fats and proteins, are preferentially utilized. Carbohydrates are used preferentially since in most individuals they are typically readily accessible, and the body will easily metabolize them for energy. Before an athletic performance to have additional energy, athletes sometimes consume some kind of high carbohydrate snack. Carbohydrates are usually utilized just a few hours after they are ingested, which is one explanation why we feed so much. Unused carbohydrates are processed or transformed into fat in the form of glycogen in the liver. The primary function of fats, by comparison, is to store energy. To brace for winter, livestock fattens up. The body usually retains the fats we consume, so the body can break down the fat stores and use them as energy if there are not enough carbohydrates accessible. Fats are metabolized somewhat gradually and it would usually require a day or two to use the fat content of a meal. This explains why people feel fuller as opposed to a low carbohydrate meal after a fatty meal. Protein, the third nutrient, is mainly used to build and replenish body materials; any surplus protein is metabolized or excreted as fuel. The body may continue to break down muscle to metabolize the protein for fuel if carbohydrate and fat reserves are exhausted. The proportion (by weight) of the three fuels used would be around 5-15% protein, 10-20% fat, and 65-85%

the carbohydrate in a traditional western diet. The body can retain some extra "fuel" as fat, or excrete it. The amount of fats in a ketogenic diet, on the other side, is substantially improved and the proportion of carbohydrates is drastically decreased. It is therefore important to monitor the overall food consumption since if the body is provided excess, it would preferentially dump the fats to revert to its preferred fuel balance. The body is forced to metabolize fat in favor of carbohydrates by limiting its overall caloric intake.

By refusing the body the carbohydrate it needs to function properly, thus pressuring it to metabolize fat, a ketogenic diet mimics a hunger or fasting condition. Ketone bodies are shaped when the fat is metabolized. It is the formation of ketone bodies that tends to play a key role in the effectiveness of a ketogenic diet. It is referred to as the body being in ketosis as the body starts making ketone bodies. Since initiating the diet, it typically takes 3 to 5 days

for the body to done ketosis. Ketosis is quickly recognizable since the ketones in the urine can be identified and can be recognized by the distinctive smell of the breath of the person. The prophylactic effects of the ketogenic diet grow with time and it will take many weeks for a ketogenic diet to have its maximum impact.

1.2. Myths about Ketogenic Diet

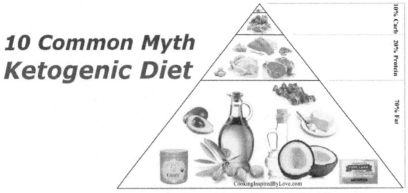

Low Carb High Fat Ketogenic Food Pyramid

A ketogenic diet is presently trending as the greatest diet for weight reduction till now. It's rich in fat and a low-carbohydrate diet that forms ketones. The effect of the breakdown of fats in the liver to be used as energy. With a keto diet numerous things are being said that is correct, but a lot of things that aren't so factual as well.

We will expose 14 myths about the keto diet below, including those linked with what to

suppose throughout the transition period, finest ratios of macros, and possible benefits

like good weight loss and mental comprehension help.

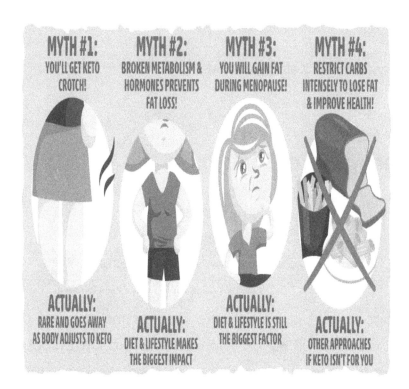

MYTH #1:
YOU'LL GET KETO CROTCH!

MYTH #2:
BROKEN METABOLISM & HORMONES PREVENTS FAT LOSS!

MYTH #3:
YOU WILL GAIN FAT DURING MENOPAUSE!

MYTH #4:
RESTRICT CARBS INTENSELY TO LOSE FAT & IMPROVE HEALTH!

ACTUALLY:
RARE AND GOES AWAY AS BODY ADJUSTS TO KETO

ACTUALLY:
DIET & LIFESTYLE MAKES THE BIGGEST IMPACT

ACTUALLY:
DIET & LIFESTYLE IS STILL THE BIGGEST FACTOR

ACTUALLY:
OTHER APPROACHES IF KETO ISN'T FOR YOU

1. The Rich in fat, rich in protein diet is Keto.

A keto diet isn't especially abundant in protein, unlike another common low-carb diet. In reality, when on a keto diet, protein consumption always must be "adequate" because this helps you to switch to ketosis and remain there. In general, so abundant protein in the diet can contribute to few of the protein being transformed to glucose until ingested, and this will be detrimental when it is about to retaining relatively low amounts of glucose. Then what proportion of protein are you going to need? A typical guideline for a ketogenic diet is to receive around 75% of the everyday calories from fat sources (for instance oils or fatty meat cuts), 5% from carbs, and 20% from protein (take or give a little is depending on the dieter). Rich-protein, low-carb diets, on the other hand, can include having 30 to 35 % (or sometimes more) of regular protein calories.

2. A Keto diet is solely a weight reduction diet.

Without any doubt over that, a ketogenic diet would promote successful weight loss. Although this does not mean that a keto diet should not be implemented to support a healthier weight if one of the goals is not good weight management. By widely encouraging metabolic fitness, for example, healthy body composition, the effects of keto will achieve a good degree of balanced mental results beyond weight advantages. Will you gain weight from a keto diet? It is perhaps possible, particularly if you do not properly embrace the diet and may not have ketosis. It is commonly accepted that if calorie intake is lower than needed by someone, Regardless of the type of diet anyone follows, weight loss will always a result in fact, from where

the calories come.

The key point? If we eat more calories daily than we do, if the source of calories is protein or fats, then you may notice the scale creeping up.

3. Claims for health care are simply claims. There's also no research.

This can't have been farther from the facts! In 1920, Johns Hopkins Medical Center doctors first established a ketogenic diet. At that moment, hundreds of experiments have studied the

impact of the diet.

4. You can't perform the workout on Keto.

For everyone, counting those on a ketogenic diet, exercising is helpful. At the start, during the workout, you feel that your energy decreases, but this would disperse as the body changes.

A ketogenic diet does not appear to trigger any loss in efficiency for most individuals, particularly in the middle of high-intensity workouts; in reality, some report getting even extra energy because the fats for fuel can be used by the body effectively. Make sure you eat sufficient calories in total and lots of fat to sustain your exercises. And if you still fail to remain active when on a diet, consider raising your carbohydrates, a little and/or attempting a more "improved ketogenic diet."

5. On the ketogenic diet and keto lifestyle, you will lose body mass.

On a keto diet, will you grow muscle? There's some proof that you can, yeah. This is how it might be a perfect way to help muscle building and boost resilience by mixing a ketogenic diet with strength-training. And keto diet does not, on its own, induce more muscle mass loss like any other diet, until you reduce calories.

6. The same thing goes with ketoacidosis & ketosis.

The two of them are very distinct and would not be mistaken. Ketoacidosis is observed as a severe diabetic problem that arises when excess ketones are produced by the body (or we can say blood acids). However, ketosis is a physiological condition in which much of the food for the body is produced by fat.

7. During their transition period, everybody faces such things.

Each person responds very differently to a ketogenic diet, so it's difficult to judge

 what you might come across. Some persons smoothly move into ketosis, while others do not.

Although these encounters may at first be unpleasant, it is usual for them to go out after one

or two weeks, so be optimistic. Through eating a "well balanced" ketogenic diet, consume

adequate water, sodium, and electrolytes (such as magnesium or potassium, like as from a

Ketogenic Multi and vegetables), fiber, you will further minimize the discomfort you feel,

 might be in supplementing with exogenous ketones (which is the form of Keto Fire).

8. On the keto, you will still have little sugar.

Some feel that their vitality and focus gets a boost as they adapt to be in ketosis. Ketones are doing a better job by supplying a constant supply of food to the brain, but staying in ketosis (and adding keto-friendly vitamins) will benefit by encouraging mental clarity, concentration, and a healthy mindset.

9. You can only remain for a brief amount of time on the keto.

In general speaking, it is advised that if you start a keto diet the first time, you continue the diet for around 2 to 3 months, and then stop for a while. Offer your body some weeks to adjust and, if it fits well for you, hop right on the ketogenic diet. Depending on how you feel, you might want to comfortably move in or out of the ketosis for several months or years. You can still contact a health provider, though. A ketogenic diet has no fixed time limit; it's just about finding out what fits better for you with your routine and objectives.

10. Occasionally, you can cheat while on keto

It may not be reasonable to ask you to adhere 100% to a keto diet. But dissimilar other diets, where it is possible to allow "cheat days" to offer you a pause and also promote your metabolism, your ketosis might shift out while cheating on the keto diet. If it's deliberate, this must not be a concern. As far as we know it's going on and you change your diet consequently, cycling a ketogenic diet out here is all right. If you notice that because of "cheating" and growing your carb consumption, you are no longer in ketosis, so by increasing your fats and reducing your carbohydrates, you will easily take some days to get back in.

11. On a keto diet, you can consume some form of fat, equivalent to common low-carb diets.

Because a keto diet isn't just about good weight loss, as compared to any forms of fatty foodstuffs, healthy fats are promoted. Many persons on a keto diet, for example, tend to eliminate high-fat fatty meat items such as bacon or pork, poor-quality sausage, and salami.

Continue to "eat clean" if you need the best out of the diet; skip trans-fats, refined goods produced from poor-quality vegetable oils, most fried foods, fast food, cheeses, and meats of questionable quality. Choose safe and cold-pressed oils (such as coconut oil or natural olive), butter, grass-fed and beef, pasture-raised livestock, wild-caught seafood, and cage-free eggs to acquire your fats from safe sources.

12. For women and men, Keto is the same.

Overall, compared with males, women incline to be more susceptible to dietary shifts and weight. It's always feasible for the women to adopt a keto diet successfully and, if they prefer, to observe intermittent fasting, however, they can do so more cautiously.

In addition to a ketogenic diet, it is advised that women concentrate on consuming a nutritious, alkaline diet, ensuring they include plenty of vegetables that are non-starchy to ensure that they receive adequate nutrients & electrolytes. Ideally, the diet can be approached in different steps, initially concentrating on full alkaline foods before including the keto component & fasting. Women can, therefore, as far as possible, decrease such causes of tension and still, pay attention to their bodies. If you are a woman adopting a keto diet, do concentrate on how your outlook & energy are affected by exercise, and what amount of sleep you get every night, the exposure of sunlight you get, the consumption of caffeine alcohol, etc.

13. When on a keto diet, intermittent fasting must take place.

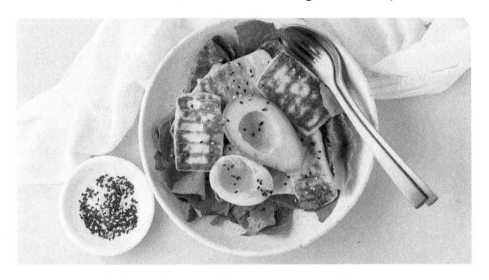

During a keto diet, intermittent fasting (known as IMF) is recommended and can help speed up outcomes (like detoxification and moving towards the weight loss goals), although it is not a necessity for ketosis to be reached or sustained. When adopting a keto diet, many individuals observe IMF to be simpler as ketosis is proven to help minimize cravings and to help sustain a regular, balanced appetite. If you are a bit hungry, not just because during a keto diet you consume plenty of gratifying fats, fiber from vegetables, and moderate protein, it happens due to ketones which help to curb appetite, so you will notice that fasting will not be

tough as it would otherwise be.

14. While on keto, you can't consume alcohol.

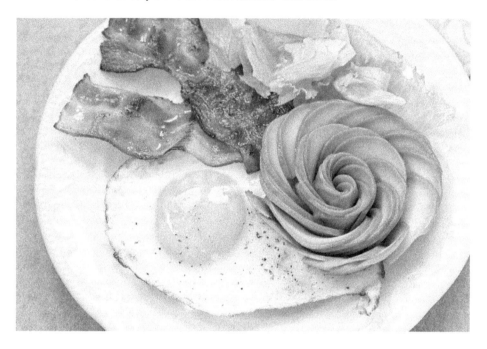

Although on the ketogenic diet, some people still prefer to drink alcohol in a balanced amount, particularly hard liquor & organic red wine. The aim is to sustain a small amount of alcohol consumption and to drink alcohol with a portion of food containing lots of fat and a certain amount of protein.

Beverages that are rich in carbs and sugar are not healthy options, such as sugar blended drinks and most breweries. If consuming alcohol allows sugar levels of blood to increase too high, and it makes it too tough to remain in ketosis, so to make a keto diet work for you, you may need to limit or eliminate alcohol.

1.4. Benefits of Ketogenic Diet

The ketogenic regimen is encircled by different controversies. Supporters of the ketogenic diet state that it is a phenomenal diet whereas rivals criticize the diet because of misconceptions about the functioning involved. As with so many questions of controversies, the truth is somewhere in between. Like most dietetic methods, a ketogenic diet has also almost no disadvantages but numerous benefits, which are as under.

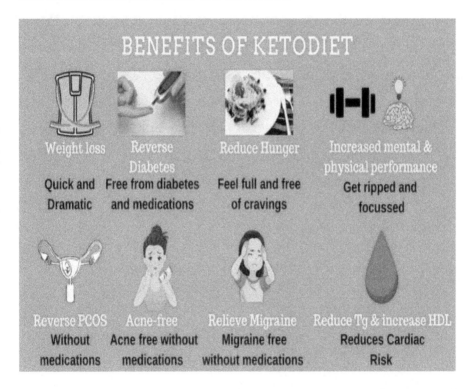

Let's have a peek at the carbohydrate pathway before exploring the advantages of the Ketogenic diet. Carbohydrates are absorbed and stored easily. Digestion begins in the mouth, as soon as the food is chewed, amylase (Such enzymes that digest carbohydrates) in the saliva now performing on the carbohydrates. In the stomach, carbohydrates are more broken down and are straightaway absorbed, once it goes into the small intestines. Carbohydrates immediately buildup the sugar level in the blood. This encourages the instant release of insulin.

High sugar level generates the release of high levels of insulin. This hormone causes the sugar to be deposited instantly in the body tissues to reduce the level of blood. Those issues can be insulin resistance when it is continually exposed to it at high levels. As the body tends to speedily stock the carbohydrates, it leads to obesity. Diabetes and cardiovascular disease can result from this cycle. The body behaves more like a fat burner than a carbohydrate-based mechanism. Analysis indicates that a carbohydrate-rich diet is the emergence of a variety of diseases, such as insulin resistance and diabetes.

1.4.1. Diabetes

A ketogenic diet that is known for rich in fats and low in carbohydrates has been found to play a vital role in decreasing and improving specific medical illnesses. It is designated as a part of the cure plan. Carbohydrates are the main source of diabetes. By cutting back on the ingestion in a ketogenic diet, the blood sugar level can be controlled. Other diabetes treatment plans work better in combination with this diet.

1.4.2. Weight Loss

A ketogenic diet has found an obvious position in the conventional dieting trend. It is now part of many fitness or dieting regimen, due to its observed effects of promoting weight loss. Initially, the idea of reducing weight with a rich fat diet upraised many eyebrows and many questions. Over time and as more satisfactory results appeared, a ketogenic diet is now slowly being incorporated as part of weight reduction plans. Carbohydrates lead to gain weight more than fats do. Remember, as we discussed above, that the hormones of insulin help the storage of

carbohydrates so that the weight will be gain. Removing or keeping the carbohydrate consumption to the least can result in considerable weight loss over time.

1.4.3. Cardiovascular Disease

A rich fat diet can be good for health. It depends on the kind and source of fats. Clean and saturated fats in the diet can keep the ingestion of carbohydrates low and improves the body's fat profile. This diet raises the HDL (which is the good cholesterol) levels and takes down the triglyceride levels. This type of fat profile is related to improve the protection against heart strokes and other cardiovascular problems.

1.4.4. Epilepsy

For a certain reason, epileptic attacks are reduced when an individual is on a ketogenic diet. This is the main reason why a ketogenic diet has been introduced. Pediatric epileptic cases are the utmost responsive to this diet. Some kids even have seizure exclusion after a few years of following the ketogenic diet while adult epilepsy has inadequate responses. The children need to fast for a limited day before the beginning of a ketogenic diet plan as a cure for epilepsy.

1.4.5. Cancer

Continuing research shows the potential that a ketogenic diet pushes cancer into reduction. It literally "famishes cancer" to reduce the indications.

1.4.6. Alzheimer's disease

Research illustrates that memory function progresses when a patient with Alzheimer's follows a ketogenic diet. They recover a few of their thought and memory functions.

1.4.7. Neurological disorders

Parkinson's disease and amyotrophic lateral sclerosis (In short ALS) are certain neurological syndromes that benefit from a ketogenic diet. The diet offers mitochondrial support in affected nerves. In this way, the symptoms improve.

1.4.8. Reverse PCOS

One frequently investigated question? Whether keto diet is a good eating technique to help manage PCOS? Different extent of life can be upset due to polycystic ovary syndrome. With other issues, PCOS can also impact weight, and numerous queries come up as to what are the suitable way to cure PCOS via diet. PCOS may be cure with medical treatments such as birth control drugs. But life routine management, such as reducing even a slight weight, might also help lessen the symptoms.

And here's a keto diet question list comes up. That's what needs to know about how a keto can affect PCOS symptoms. The keto diet is a nutritional strategy that emphasizes reducing carbs and taking a high amount of fat so that body uses the fat in energy form. Individuals on the ketogenic diet typically haven't more than 50 grams of carbs per day. As carbs change into glucose in the body, so insulin is required to bring that sugar to the cells to get energy. Like, on the ketogenic diet, the person needs to limit the carb intake, which can assist to relieve the insulin resistance which might occur as an outcome of having PCOS. Also, losing weight and insulin levels can help some women to resume normal ovulation and better fertility.

1.4.9. Efficient against fighting with metabolic syndrome

The possibility of developing diabetes and cardiac failure is typically correlated with metabolic syndrome. Metabolic syndrome contains signs such as:

Abdominal obesity,

High level of blood Pressure

Excessive amounts of sugar in the blood

High level of triglycerides

A low-carbohydrate diet can be successful in maintaining both of these effects, but a keto diet can help hold metabolic syndrome away and can even help reduce weight without bariatric surgery. These symptoms may be removed by adopting the keto diet schedule.

Chapter 2: Menopause and Ketogenic Diet

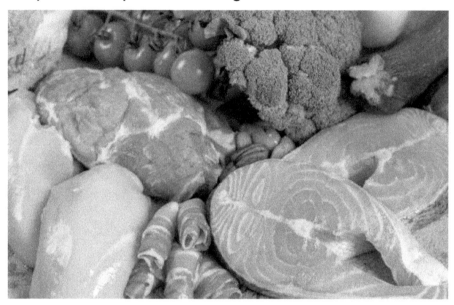

The indicators of menopause can be disturbing for many women. The weight increase, hot flashes, changes in the skin, lack of sleep, low libido, annoyance, and mood fluctuations unsurprisingly happen during this phase. These symptoms can make one feel extremely concerned about the health and well-being. Luckily, we can manage these tough symptoms with healthy habits, starting with the diet. These side effects of menopause are caused by inequities in sex hormones (estrogen and testosterone). A ketogenic diet can help balance these hormones and potentially improve menopause symptoms. In this section, we discuss how we can use a ketogenic diet to manage the symptoms if we're going through menopause.

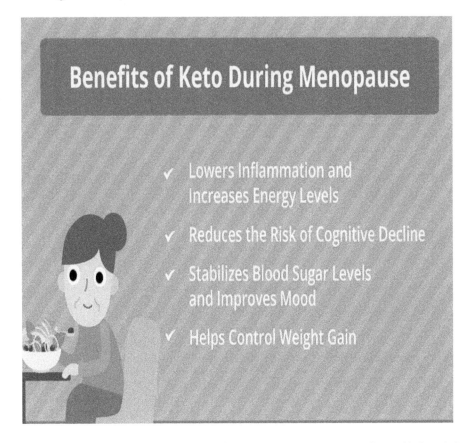

Benefits of Keto During Menopause

✓ Lowers Inflammation and Increases Energy Levels

✓ Reduces the Risk of Cognitive Decline

✓ Stabilizes Blood Sugar Levels and Improves Mood

✓ Helps Control Weight Gain

Menopause procedure begins when a woman hasn't had her menstrual period for over twelve months. It usually happens in women over the age of 50 and it is a mark that all of her available eggs have been down. Due to which, estrogen and testosterone, the reproductive hormone level drops. These hormonal changes can generate metabolic difficulties and unwanted symptoms, such as insulin resistance, glucose intolerance, high BP, weight gain, hot flashes, night sweats, loss of libido, and so on so forth. This occurs because all the hormones in the body are linked. Therefore, when the level of reproductive hormones drops, insulin also gets affected, causing metabolic changes. The reduction in testosterone drops the body's ability to build new muscle mass and slowing down the metabolism even more. A reduction in muscle mass and insulin issues leads to fat gain, mainly around your stomach, Inflammation, and oxidative stress, speeding up the aging procedure, encouraging even more weight gain. Auspiciously, adopting a healthy diet that particularly stimulates hormonal balance is one of the coolest ways to improve insulin resistance, maintain muscle mass, lessening inflammation, and maintain a healthy weight. A ketogenic diet, a low carbohydrate, rich in fat diet, has been recognized to diminish a lot of the metabolic issues that happen during menopause because it helps to balance hormones.

2.1. Six ways to improve menopause through keto

A high-fat, low carbohydrate strategy is a ketogenic diet. It's not new, but in recent years, as low-fat, high-carb diets have been seen to be the true culprits behind America's epidemic of obesity, heart disease, and diabetes, it has gained considerable momentum. The new study is being conducted to discover all the possible health benefits, including hormonal factors, with a revived public interest in a ketogenic diet for health and weight loss.

Here are 6 explanations why during menopause a ketogenic diet is beneficial:

1: The Control of Insulin

While no detailed trials have been performed on the complications of keto and menopause, we will learn a lot about the hormonal impact of keto from studies on women with the polycystic ovarian syndrome (PCOS). We've discovered from this analysis that insulin and sex hormones are intricately related. Studies have shown that with a ketogenic diet, normalizing insulin levels can help get sex hormones back into equilibrium, reducing symptoms such as weight gain in women with PCOS. This suggests that you will also regulate sex hormones by raising insulin levels by low carb, high fat diet, and therefore have a decrease in typical menopause symptoms. The influence that keto has on insulin allows it an effective diet to regulate sex hormones and to manage symptoms of menopause.

2: Lose weight

One of the main problems of many women after menopause is weight gain. They may appear to be doing all right, but they are still adding weight The bottom line is that low amounts of estrogen induce weight gain, and it appears to accumulate in the abdominal region in particular. For females who were used to wearing a certain pant size, this may ring warning bells and now nothing matches. They will also continue to cut calories to reduce weight, but this will cause some menopausal symptoms worse. Low-calorie diets delay the metabolism, first of all. They also worsen muscle and bone mass deterioration, increasing the probability of osteoporosis. In itself, menopause often induces muscle and bone deterioration, so why make things worse by consuming a low-calorie diet? The ketogenic diet may be a fantastic way to control weight once you feel the pounds piling up. Evidence suggests that a high-fat diet and low carbs will help women drop weight and hold it off. In a 2015 report, low carbohydrate or low-fat diet was asked to follow postmenopausal women who endured breast cancer. In six months, those who adopted the low-carb diet dropped 23.1 pounds, 7.6 percent body weight, and 3.7 inches in their waist. Although both groups lost weight, substantially more was lost by the low carb group. There are many explanations that a keto diet leads to weight management and can make it easier for women during menopause to sustain a healthier weight. Larger consumption of protein improves satiety. You're less inclined to overeat when you feel complete and satisfied. In comparison, the reduction of most carbohydrates also results in reduced calorie consumption overall. A ketogenic diet regulates the chemicals of starvation. A 2013 research discovered that participants had healthy amounts of ghrelin after 8 weeks on a ketogenic diet. In certain carb-based diets, ghrelin is an appetite-stimulating hormone that enhances desire. Subjects have lost 13% of their body weight in the same sample and had lower overall hunger ratings. Keto accelerates digestion and the burning of calories. Several calories are absorbed by gluconeogenesis, or by the processing of glucose from non-carb compounds. Metabolism is often accelerated by lipolysis or the breakdown of fat for energy. Any diet that speeds up the metabolism would be helpful for women who suffer a metabolic slowdown. The bottom line is that some of the weight gain encountered in menopause can help stave off the ketogenic diet and may help normalize metabolism.

3: Hot Flashes Elimination

Hot flashes are an exceedingly annoying menopause complication. They will interrupt your sleep and make you feel very unpleasant. While the precise cause of hot flashes is not understood, low estrogen levels and their influence on the hypothalamus is presumably linked to them, a part of the brain that controls body temperature. Ketone bodies formed during ketosis can help protect the brain and minimize inflammation, which can help to control the temperature of the body.

4: Regulation between Sex Hormones

Because of such fluctuating hormones, lack of libido can be one side effect of menopause. A high-fat diet will, therefore, serve to boost both the levels of estrogen and testosterone, contributing to raising libido. Sex hormones are manufactured from fat. It was seen to decrease circulating sex hormones after a low-fat diet and may in turn decrease libido. Research has also shown the reverse, that in women, consuming a higher fat diet increases sexual function. Consuming a high-fat, ketogenic diet provides the body the raw materials it requires to sustain quantities of sex hormones, an essential component in sustaining a stable menopausal libido

5: High energy levels

In terms of energy levels, ketogenic diets may also help. There are no longer big swings of blood sugar that induce energy declines as the body switches to using fat for energy instead of carbohydrates. Your body also now has an almost infinite supply of calories (your fat stores) to tap into, growing the energy levels anytime it wants to.

6: Great Sleep, Better Sleep

During menopause, following a ketogenic diet will even boost sleep. Healthy sleep would be a great symptom, due to the elimination of hot flashes, better blood sugar control, healthier weight, and hormone balance. It's time to put it into effect now that you know how a ketogenic diet will better relieve the effects of menopause and boost your general wellbeing.

Chapter 3: Do's and Don'ts of Ketogenic Diet

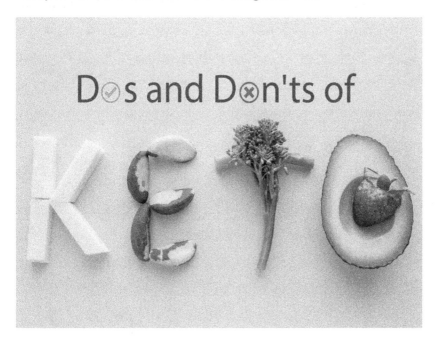

Among individuals with health & wellness aspirations, weight reduction, blood glucose regulation, and increased athletic efficiency, a ketogenic diet has become a common alternative. You might make errors that keep you from completing ketosis if you're new to the diet.

We're going to teach you in this book how to successfully execute the diet with our collection of dos and don'ts. To keep on track, you may also want this list. Continue to learn.

3.1. Do's of Keto diet

1. Prepare the food list for a ketogenic diet.

What should I consume with this keto diet? "If you ever catch yourself posing this question, reading a collection of ketogenic approved recipes would aid. Keep for diets that are rich in fat and low carbohydrates. Fatty meat pieces, plants, eggs & dairy are examples. Keep your products and preparations basic, since it requires time to adapt to the diet. You shouldn't be scared to try as long as we satisfy the micronutrient & macronutrient requirements.

2. Take a full meal.

It is a fact that there are a lot of processed snacks that make them easy to consume. Packaged drugs, though, can include poor fats and sugars that come with different labels, such as Agave Nectar, Maltodextrin, Dextran, and more. The way to maintain optimal quality is by consuming foods in their usual state. Whole foods, which help avoid micronutrient malnutrition, are abundant in minerals & vitamins. Choose minimally processed foods instead, if you're particularly busy.

3. Eat lots of healthy fat.

This mistake is made by several keto dieters; they consume extra fat but do not pay heed to the quality of the fats. Although having 60-75 percent of the calories from the fats is essential, you have to make it clear that calories come from polyunsaturated fats & good monounsaturated and Note that there is typically a healthy form of fat present in seafood, nuts, beans, and vegetables. Sardines, walnuts, Salmon, pecans, lettuce, flaxseed, and avocados are several examples.

4. Check the levels of blood glucose.

Keto aims to bring the body into a condition of ketosis. You should maintain the glucose of blood under control (approx. less than 100 mg/dL) for you to do it.

Watching for fluctuations in the sugar levels when you're doing keto makes sense. This is particularly valid if you attempt alternative "keto" diets, encounter tension, or evaluate the efficacy of fasting. It is therefore recommended for patients with type 2 diabetes to observe the blood glucose periodically.

5. Lookout for sugars that are concealed.

Done all the prescribed by the keto routine, but don't see results Maybe you deal with an adversary, secret carbohydrates. It doesn't mean that you're in ketosis simply because you're skipping rice, noodles, and pastries.

Several fat-free dressings appear to be full of sugar. Coleslaw, Greek yogurt, Sauces, condiments, and cashew nuts are certain types of secret carbohydrates. Amazed? To prevent these secret carbohydrates, the easiest option is to prepare your food in your home.

6. Always drink plenty of fluid like water.

Ketosis is considered to cause multiple side effects. Dehydration is one of these adverse effects. Some persons urinate more often than have ketosis. This arises because glycogen stocks are decreasing in their bodies. If you don't know what actually glycogen is, it's the primary source of glucose storage. You need to improve your water consumption on keto. It would also help to stop stones in the kidney and relieve headaches by doing so. Try adding any berries, ice, or cucumbers into the water to meet the water consumption targets.

7. Take supplements containing vitamins and minerals.

On keto, should you take supplements of vitamins and minerals? The response is "indeed yes". Because you cut off several ingredients, a ketogenic diet will cause deficiencies of minerals and vitamins. Some individuals often do not adopt a well-balanced keto diet by consuming something fatty, especially bad fat. Poor fats sometimes lack nutrients. Ensure that you receive sufficiently zinc, B-complex, vitamin D, magnesium, sodium, vitamin C, and vitamins. Apart from a multivitamin supplement, select whole food.

8. Be prepare for keto flu

There's a set of symptoms that certain individuals who initiate keto encounter. These effects are recognized as "keto flu." As the body removes from carbs, keto flu arises. Headaches, dizziness, nausea, stomach cramps, and muscle weakening are the recorded signs.

Always note that people respond differently to keto. Some have and some don't have the keto flu. However, one needs to follow to reduce these symptoms: stop strenuous exercise, get enough sleep, drink sufficient water, raise good fat consumption, and substitute electrolytes.

3.2. Don'ts of Keto Diet

1. Eat food that is low in fat. Since keto is a rich-fat diet, prioritizing items that contain more fat makes sense. Research has also found that the sugar level in less-calorie items such as baked goods and dairy products is greater. It doesn't mean that they are low-sugar simply because the labels claim less-calorie." Your ketogenic diet provides multiple options to incorporate more fat. You should add cheese to your meals that are made up of vegetables. Make recipes of avocado, drizzle salads with olive oil, and use MCT oil.

2. Use underground-grown veggies.

Keto is perfect for cruciferous vegetables and those veggies which grown up on the ground. These vegetables have less sugar and are full of antioxidants and nutrients. Cauliflower, cabbage, broccoli, and spinach are low-carb choices. Onions, sweet potatoes, beets maize, peas can be prohibited.

3. Chewing so many nuts

Always remember that all nuts are equally made. As somebody on keto, for your choices and quantity of nuts, you must be cautious. Cashews, pistachios, and pine have nuts that appear to contain lots of carbs. Pecans, Brazil and macadamias, are the types of keto nuts. Always remember that while rich-carb and low-carb nuts are present, you should not go overboard with nuts in particular. It's nice to eat nuts, but when you need energy, not when you're hungry and just need anything to chew on.

4. Using the keto diet for a fast cure.

A keto diet is not an immediate effective diet. It's a mode of life, a lifestyle. We see so many individuals getting in this diet to easily lose weight and they stop immediately if they don't. Any persons, when they get keto flu, feel frustrated due to lack of study. Another myth is that ketogenic diet and low-carb are similar things. Having a better understanding of what ketosis is? Is it the easiest way to tackle keto? Know your research, your accurate macros of keto, and expect any improvements.

5. Without referring to the doctor, pursue Keto.

It will be nice to speak up about your keto diet if you see a specialist or you have a health problem (for instance, diabetes or any heart disease). Since there could be drugs that contraindicate keto, the doctor needs to know your dietetic strategy. Most notably, inform your doctor about your keto encounter. Have you gained more energy? Has the blood glucose reduced?

Hopefully, these do's and don'ts can boost the adhesion to a ketogenic diet. Choose more genuine ingredients and healthy fats to bring out the best results from the diet. Don't ignore the requirements for micronutrients. As a diet, accept keto, instead of an instant cure. Keep yourself updated.

3.3. Restricted food

To cause ketosis, carbohydrates are primarily limited. The body, however, will adjust to dietary change. Proteins, thus, and Fats, too, ought to be monitored.

- Fats

    In a ketogenic diet, fats are usually promoted. It is the predominant source of energy during ketosis. Approximately 60% to 80% of total calories are supposed to come with fats. The value depends on a ketogenic diet's target. Some can also use fats as 90% of the overall dietary intake.

    However, when deciding the kind of fats to use, there are a few rules to consider. No omega-6 polyunsaturated fats. Insignificant concentrations, omega-6 fats appear to be inflammatory.

- Corn oil
- Soy
- Cottonseed

 Stop seed or nut-based oils since they are rich in omega-6 and may hurt the body.

- Almond oil
- Flaxseeds

- Sesame Seed Oil

- Stop mayonnaise and dressings with commercial salads. If inevitable, verify the carbohydrate material.

- Stop fats and Trans fats that are hydrogenated.

  These were found to be correlated with increased risk for the production of coronary heart issues and other health complications.

- The Proteins

It is critical to select proteins since they will influence the diet over time. Steroid-treated and antibiotic-treated animals can cause problems with health. Choose grass-fed, free-range, and natural. Ignore those who have been fed with hormones, particularly RBST.

However, review the starch content that could come from the use of extenders or fillers while selecting processed meat items. Avoid any curing meat that contains honey or sugar.

- Carbohydrates

In specific, ketogenic diets impose extreme limits on the consumption of carbohydrates. The restriction is based on the level of activity of the person and level of metabolism. Generally, a net daily carbohydrate consumption of less than 50 or 60 grams is needed for a ketogenic diet. Individuals with healthy metabolism (such as athletes) can intake as many as 100 or more grams per day. It could be important for sedentary individuals with type 2 diabetes mellitus to limit carbohydrates to less than 30 grams in a day. It relies on tolerance and the state of wellbeing. The aim of a keto diet is also based on it.

- Vegetables

Although the key sources of carbohydrates in a ketogenic diet are vegetables, some need to be prevented. Some veggies have large amounts of sugar such as peppers, tomatoes, and onions. The bulk of vegetables that grow underground are starchy, producing plenty of starch.

- The Sweets

The typical sweet foods are completely avoided since they are very rich in sugars and carbohydrates. They are:

- Cakes

- Sweetbread

- Bread and buns

- Glace-fruit

- Chocolates: These contain diet chocolate and other types of chocolate, including lollipops. Biscuits: normal, iced, or chocolate-coated, with cream filling

- Pies

- Pastry

- Puddings

- Sweetened toppings and syrups

- Milk condensed

- Ice-creams

- Jam: all kinds, such as diabetic jam

- Milk flavorings

- Drinks such as Ovaltine, Milo

- Sauces

- Chutneys and pickles

- Flavored yogurt- Artificial flavoring may include sugar as malt dextrin or in any other shape.

- Cordials and sugar-containing soft beverages.

- Fruit Juice

- Chewing gum, including some who are sugarless

- Sweetened syrups and treatments for coughing

- Sugars

  Sugar is a rich carbohydrate supply that needs to be stopped. Sugar is commonly known in ways such as brown sugar, white sugar, castor, and icing. In refined foods and medicines, it may also be an element

3.4. Permitted Food

In a ketogenic diet, meals consist predominantly of 3 specific forms of food. There's a fruit, a diet high in proteins, and a source of fat.

- Fats

    The ketogenic diet calls for extra fatty fats. They may be used, such as frying or pan grilling, as part of the cooking method. Fats may also be in the form of sauces and dressings. A way of adding fats into the diet is often to simply top a slice of steak with butter. Those that are ketogenic are the better form of fat. The MCTs or medium-chain triglycerides are the best, which involve MCT oil and coconut oil. To generate ketones, these fats are readily metabolized.

    For ketosis, other healthy fats are:

- Omega-3 and Omega-6 Fatty acids

- Trout

- Salmon

- Tuna

- Shellfish

- Saturated and monounsaturated fats

- Olive oil

- Red palm-oil

- Butter

- Cheese

- Avocado

- Egg yolks

- Non-hydrogenated oil (when cooking)

- Tallow beef

- Lards that are non-hydrogenated

- Coconut oil

- High oleic acid

- Oils of Safflower

- Sunflowers oil

- Peanut-butter

- Skin of chicken

- Fat of beef

- Coconut butter

- The Proteins

In a keto diet, every form of meat is effectively permitted. The sort of cut or preparation should not differentiate.

- Pork
- Beef
- Veal
- Venison

- Lamb
- Poultry

Use every sort of poultry item. It is preferable to have the skin on since it improves the meal's fat quality. As they have high carbohydrate content, preparation does not require the use of breading and batter. Acceptable preparations are based on an individual's choice.

- Chicken
- Quail
- Turkey
- Duck
- Sea Foods

Seafood is a decent source of protein as well. Some include elevated amounts of omega-3 fatty acids, vitamins, and minerals that can help sustain proper nutrition for healthier people.

Fish has a large content of safe omega-3 fatty acids. Choose fish that are captured in the wild and places clear of mercury.

- Tuna
- Catfish
- Halibut
- Flounder
- Cod
- Snapper
- Trout
- Salmon
- Mackerel

- Shellfish
- Clams
- Squid
- Mahi-mahi
- Oysters
- Lobster
- Mussel
- Scallops
- Carbohydrates
- Vegetables

The primary sources of carbohydrates in a ketogenic diet involve vegetables. There are excellent opportunities for organically raised vegetables. There isn't much difference between organic and non-organic in terms of nutritional value. The difference lies in the risk of eating vegetables treated with dark leafy vegetables with the lowest nutritionally valuable carbohydrate content.

- Spinach
- Watercress
- Cabbage, all sorts
- Lettuce, both forms
- Kale
- Sprouts from Brussels
- Broccoli
- Celery
- Cucumber
- Cauliflower
- Bean sprout

- Radishes
- Asparagus
- Dairy and Milk Goods

In a ketogenic diet, milk and dairy items are fundamental. There is a preference for natural and renewable sources. It is often easier to select the complete fat varieties than the fat-free or reduced-fat versions. In a ketogenic diet, eggs are staples

It is a perfect source of fats and proteins.

Cheese, from hard to soft kinds. There are carbs in it. Include the cheeses in the daily carbohydrates count. Some of them are:

- Mascarpone
- Cheddar
- Mozzarella
- Cream cheese
- Cottage cheese

It is therefore advised that sour cream be used in the diet. It serves more interesting varieties.

- Nuts

In a ketogenic diet, a reasonable intake of nuts is permitted. Proteins, fats, and carbohydrates are rich in them. The Variety of Nuts needs to be observed for carbohydrate, fats, and protein ingredients and included in the regular keto estimation.

Roasted nuts and Seeds are the safest since they eliminate something in the body that may inflict damage or mess with ketosis. Nuts are mainly promoted as a snack. Almonds, macadamias, and walnuts are the right nuts for inclusion. Some nuts are high in omega-6 fatty acids, which in the body can induce inflammation. Pistachio and cashew produce higher carbohydrate levels. Best to slowly rack these up.

- Spices

It may be tough to adapt to fewer carbohydrate consumption within the first several weeks after adopting a ketogenic diet. Individuals who have the sweet tooth can find it too hard to handle in their cravings. People that are used to consuming meals of high carbohydrates such as spaghetti and pasta or processed foods can complain of boring meals that are less tasty. After some time, ketogenic foods will become boring.   Spices can spice things up.   You may add fresh and dried spices to the meals and also beverages to make the meals a little more tempting and entertaining. Spices have carbohydrates. Few spices should include in daily carbs and ketogenic count. Typically, pre-made spice mixes include added sugar. To add the accurate amount of total carbohydrates, count, one should read the labels of the content

This is the form of sugar that should be avoided in a ketogenic diet. Not just for the tastes, but also for the different health benefits that they bring, spices may be included. Some of these advantageous spices Includes:

- Basil
- Black pepper
- Cayenne pepper

- Cilantro
- Cinnamon
- Dust of chili
- Cumin
- Parsley
- Oregano
- Sage
- Rosemary
- Turmeric
- Thyme
- Sweeteners

In curbing cravings for food and sweets, artificial sweeteners are beneficial. They lead to achieving progress in adhering to a Ketogenic diet. Using chemical sweeteners such as Stevia and E-Z Sweets is safest. Carbohydrate count does not impact them. When sweeteners, since no binders such as dextrose and maltodextrin have been

added, the liquid form is preferred.

Some of the suggested sweeteners are listed below:

- Sucralose (the liquid form is recommended)
- Xylitol
- Erythritol
- Monk fruits
- The Beverages

The low ingestion of carbohydrates in the body has a diuretic impact. Carbohydrates draw water into them, leading to the retention of water by lowering the carbohydrates in the diet, a very little amount of water is retained and more is excreted.

This may render a person predisposed to dehydration. It is a necessity to consume sufficient volumes of water daily. The likelihood of diseases of the urinary tract and bladder discomfort often rises as the body is losing more water.

The low ingestion of carbohydrates in the body has a diuretic impact. Carbohydrates draw water into them, leading to the retention of water. By lowering the carbohydrates in the diet, a very little amount of water is retained and more is excreted. This may render a person predisposed to dehydration. It is a necessity to consume sufficient volumes of water daily. The likelihood of diseases of the urinary tract and bladder discomfort often rises as the body is losing more water.

Drink more than the normal regular consumption of 8 glasses of water suggested. To increase, the hydration status, add other forms of beverages. Coffee and tea can also be added to daily liquid intake. Only coffee and tea do not affect the ketosis but the added ingredients into it will work for sure. Choose artificial sweeteners. Whether, drink full-cream coffee or tea and omit all the sugar together. Instead of fruit smoothies, power smoothies or protein shakes are better to use. Sugars that may inhibit ketosis are found in the fruits.

- Vegetable juice

When on a ketogenic diet, using the permitted vegetable forms is also great to drink ideas.

Chapter 4: Keto Meal Plan

Planning is important for progress on a ketogenic diet. This chapter of the book will show you how to make a meal idea for a ketogenic diet to fit your needs and objectives.

We have broken it down into five stages to help you build the right meal idea for yourself.

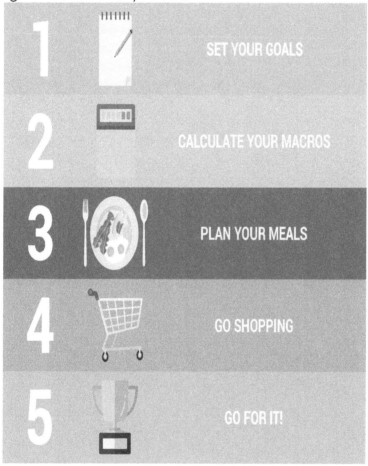

1. Set the goal

What is the purpose of consuming a ketogenic diet for you? Think of the outcomes you'd like to achieve, whether it's weight reduction, improved emotional clarity, avoidance of illness, or better physical wellbeing. Write them down somewhere the day you see them. It would help to adapt your meal plans to your needs with this in mind beforehand, as well as making it easy to adhere to your keto diet.

2. Evaluate the macros

On a ketogenic diet, macronutrient levels are very important. On a ketogenic diet, consider the macro ratios. Based on your body composition and lifestyle,

working from here will allow you to decide whether and how much of each category to consume.

3. Plan the meal

Planning what you'll consume depends on your regular macros! You could be preparing for a few days or at a time for the entire week. Most keto recipes have a list macro breakdown so you don't have to quantify it. You can check ingredients to a diet app if they don't, for their macros and calorie count.

Decide which meals each day you'll get. On a sheet of paper, it helps to list them out. Consider that:

How many people can eat the meals in your home (or how many servings you'll need to make)

How you like each day to be planned. Do you intend on having breakfast, for instance, or are you already going to have lunch and dinner most days?

When your meals are set, make a grocery list for each meal with the items you'll need. The ingredients are grouped by types, such as "meat," "dairy," "vegetables," etc.

Time to go to the grocery now!

4. Go on a shopping

A simple rule of thumb: buy first the perimeter of the store. That's where they place fresh fruit, poultry, and milk goods.

The internal aisles for oils and other specific keto stuff will need to be visited, but shopping on the outside first eliminates overwhelm, lets you concentrate on the healthiest items, and makes it easier to avoid some junky processed stuff that is surely not keto-friendly (out of sight, out of mind).

5. Go for it,

Your ingredients are yours. You've planned the meals Perhaps most of your meals ought to be

made and cooked ahead of time and stored for quik grab 'N go.

4.2. Keto Diet grocery list

Here we list out those items which should be needed to start the keto process.

4.2.1 List of Week 1

Meat

- Thick-cut pork, 24 strips
- Beef, ground (80% lean)-30 ounces
- Thighs of chicken, boneless-2 pounds
- Eggs-17 large-sized
- Ham, delicatessen, sliced-3 ounces
- Ham, 6 ounces' fat-free
- Salmon, boneless-4 fillets (6-ounce)

Vegetables and Fruits

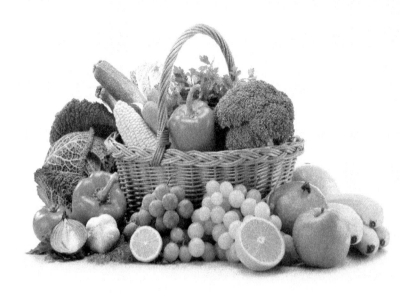

- 1 bunch of asparagus

- Avocado- 3 thin, 3 medium-sized

- Beets: 1 tiny beet

- Bell pepper, red—1 small, 1 small

- Cauliflower- 2 cups

- Chives- 1 bunch of chives

- Cucumber, English-Medium 1 1/2

- Garlic- 1 head

- Kale: 1 cup

- Lemon-1

- 5 cups of lettuce

- Mushrooms-1 cup

- Onion, red—1 tiny, 1 small

- Onion, yellow—1 short, 1 medium

- Spinach - 2 cups

- Tomatoes -1/2 cup of tomatoes

- Zucchini: 1 tiny, 1 wide

Frozen and Refrigerated Products

- Unsweetened almond milk- 1 3/4 cups

- Blueberries, 1/4 cup frozen

- Cheddar cheese, shredded-1 3/4 cups

- Unsweetened coconut milk, 1 cup

- 9 ounces' cream cheese

- Strong cream-1/4 cup

- Mayonnaise- 3 teaspoons of mayonnaise

- Parmesan ham rubbed—1 cup

- Provolone cheese, 1/4 cup shredded

- Sour cream: 1 cup

- Yogurt, full-fat-3/4 cup

Staples and Dry Products Pantry

- Almonds, whole, 1 cup

- 1 cup plus 1 tablespoon of almond butter

- 1/2 cup almond flour

- Vinegar with apple cider

- Basil pesto-1/4 cup

- Black pepper

- Soup, beef, 3 cups

- Chia seeds—1 teaspoon

- Powder of Chili

- Powder of chocolate, unsweetened

- 1/4 cup coconut flour

- Coconut Oil

- Tartar milk

- Mustard from Dijon

- Ground cinnamon •

- Ground Cumin •

- Olive Oil

- Liquid extract of stevia

- 16 macadamia nuts

- Paprika

- Erythritol dried

- Protein powder, white egg, vanilla-1/4 cup

- Pumpkin bread cinnamon spice

- Seasoning ranch

- Salt

- Tomato paste- 2 teaspoons of the paste

4.2.2 List of Week 2

Meat

- Thick-cut pork, 19 strips

- Thighs of chicken, boneless-2 pounds

- Eggs - 26 large eggs

- Ham, delicatessen, diced-1/4 cup

- Ham, free of fat: 2 pounds plus 1 ounce

- Tenderloin of bacon, boneless-1 1/2 pounds

- Salmon, boneless - 8 ounces

- Tuna, ahi-4 steaks (6-ounce)

Vegetables and Fruits

- Avocado- 2 short, 2 medium

- Green bell pepper, 1 tiny

- Cauliflower: three cups

- Celery- 1 tiny stalk

- Garlic- 1 head

- 1 bit of ginger

- Green beans, 2 cups

- Lemon-1

- Lettuce-4 1/4 cups

- Onion, red—1 tiny, 1 small

- Onion, purple, 1 tiny

- 1 bunch of parsley

- Rosemary-one bunch

- 4 ounces spring greens

- Tomato- 1 tiny tomato

Frozen and Refrigerated Products

- Almond oil, an unsweetened-3⁄4 cup of milk

- Butter - 1 tablespoon of butter

- Cream cheese, 1 ounce

- 1 cup plus 1 tablespoon heavy cream

- Mayonnaise- 3 teaspoons of mayonnaise

- Parmesan, 1/4 cup shaved

- Staples and Dry Products Pantry

- Almond butter: 1 3⁄4 cups

- 2 1⁄2 cups almond flour

- Baking Powder

- Black pepper

- Broth, chicken-five cups

- 1/2 cup of Chia seeds

- Bouillon of chicken-4 cubes

- Paste with chili garlic

- Powder of chocolate, unsweetened

- 2 teaspoons of coconut flour

- Coconut oil, canned-3 1/4 cups

- Coconut Oil

- Tartar milk

- Dijon Mustard

- 2 scoops of egg white protein powder (40g)

- Garam masala

- Ground cinnamon

- Ground Nutmeg

- Guar gum

- Olive Oil

- Powder of Onion

- Liquid extract of stevia

- Pine nuts, 1/3 cup roasted

- Erythritol dried

- Vinegar from red wine

- Salt

- Sesame beans, black-1/4 cup

- Sesame beans, toasted-1/2 cup

- Sesame beans, white-1/4 cup

- Smoked paprika

- 3 tbsp. tomato paste

- Extract of vanilla

- Sesame oil

- Soy sauce

- Extract of vanilla

4.3. Keto Diet Pyramid

Essential fatty
acids support the
cardiovascular,
reproductive, immune
and nervous systems.

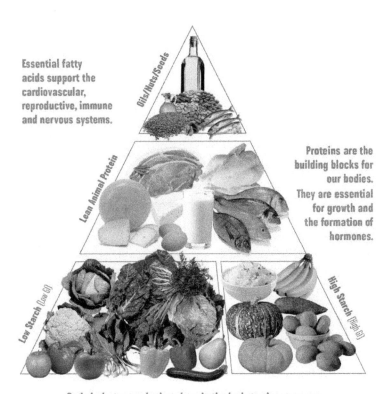

Proteins are the
building blocks for
our bodies.
They are essential
for growth and
the formation of
hormones.

Carbohydrates are broken down in the body to give us energy.

Chapter 5: Ketogenic diet meal recipes.

5.1. Recipes for breakfast

1. Veggies and Parmesan with Sheet Pan Eggs
Servings: 6 Servings:

Prep Time: 5 minutes

Cooking time: 15 minutes

Ingredients:

- 12 big, whisked eggs

- Salt and pepper

- 1 tiny red pepper, diced

- 1 tiny yellow, chopped onion

- 1 cup of diced mushrooms

- 1 cup of zucchini diced

- 1 cup of Parmesan cheese freshly grated

Instructions:

1. Preheat the oven to 350 ° F and then grease a rimmed baking sheet with cooking spray.

2. In a cup, whisk the eggs until frothy with salt and pepper.

3. Stir in the tomatoes, mushrooms, onions, and zucchini until well combined.

4. In the baking pan, pour the mixture and scatter it into an even layer.

5. Sprinkle with parmesan and bake until the egg is set, for 12 to 15 minutes.

6. Let it cool slowly, then slice it into serving squares.

Nutrition Info: 215 calories, 14g of fat, 18.5g of protein, 5g of carbohydrates, 1g of fiber, 4g of net carbohydrates.

2. Tomato Mozzarella Egg Muffins
Servings: 12 Servings:

Time to prep: 5 minutes

Cook Time: Twenty-five minutes

Ingredients:

- 1 tablespoon of butter

- 1 tomato medium, finely diced

- 1/2 cup of yellow onion diced

- 12 big, whisked eggs

- 1/2 cup of coconut milk canned

- 1/4 cup of green onion cut

- Salt and pepper

- 1 cup of mozzarella cheese shredded

Instructions:

1. Preheat the oven to 350 ° F and grease the pan with cooking spray.

2. In a medium skillet over medium heat, melt the butter.

3. Put the tomatoes and onions in the pan and cook until tender, for 3 to 4 minutes.

4. Pour the mixture into muffin cups.

5. Combine the eggs, coconut milk, green onions, salt, and pepper, and mix properly. Then put a spoon in the muffin cup.

6. Sprinkle with cheese, then bake until the egg is set, for 20 to 25 minutes.

Nutrition Information: 135 calories, 10.5g of fat, 9g of protein, 2g of carbohydrates, 0.5g of fiber, 1.5g of carbohydrates.

3. Cinnamon & Almond Porridge
Servings: 1 Serving:

Prep time: 5 minutes

Cook time: 5 minutes

Ingredients:

- 1 tablespoon of butter

- 1 tablespoon of coconut flour

- 1 large egg, whisked

- 1/8 teaspoon cinnamon powder

- Pinch of salt

- 1/4 cup of canned coconut milk

- 1 almond butter tablespoon

Instructions:

1. In a medium saucepan over a low flame, melt the butter.

2. Put the coconut flour, egg, cinnamon, and salt and whisk.

3. While whisking, add the coconut milk and stir in the almond butter until well smooth.

4. Simmer over low heat, stirring regularly, until fully heated.

5. Spoon and serve in a bowl.

Nutrition Information: 470 calories, 42g of fat, 13g of protein, 15g of carbohydrates, 8g of fiber, 7g of net carbohydrates

4. Crispy Chai Waffles
Servings: 4 Servings:

Prep time: 10 minutes

Cook time: 20 minutes

Ingredients:

- Four large eggs separated into whites and yolks

- 3 teaspoons of coconut flour

- 3 teaspoons erythritol powder

- 1 1/4 teaspoon baking powder

- 1 teaspoon Vanilla extract

- 1/2 teaspoon ground cinnamon

- 1/4 teaspoon of ground ginger

- Ground cloves pinch

- Cardamom ground pinch

- 3 teaspoons of molten coconut oil

- 3 teaspoons almond milk unsweetened

Instructions:

1. Separate the eggs into two separate bowls.

2. Whip the egg whites until they stiff peaks and put aside.

3. Whisk the coconut flour with the egg yolks, erythritol, baking powder,

add vanilla, cinnamon, cardamom, and cloves in another bowl.

4. When whisking, apply the molten coconut oil to the second bowl and whisk

in almond milk.

5. Fold the egg whites carefully until they're combined.

6. Grease the preheated waffle iron with cooking spray.

7. Spoon 1/2 cup or so of batter onto the iron.

8. Cook the waffle according to directions from the maker.

9. Remove the waffle to a plate and repeat with the batter that remains.

Nutrition Information: 215 calories, 17g of fat, 8g of protein, 8g of carbohydrates,

4g of fiber, 4g of net weight,

5. Sheet Pan Eggs with Ham and Pepper Jack

Servings: 6 Servings:

Time to prep: 5 minutes

Cook time: 15 minutes

Ingredients:

- 12 big, whisked eggs

- Salt and pepper

- Two cups of sliced ham

- 1 cup of shredded cheese and pepper jack

Instructions:

1. Preheat the oven to 350 ° F and cook a rimmed baking sheet with oil.

2. In a cup, whisk the eggs until frothy with salt and pepper.

3. Stir in the cheese and ham once well mixed.

4. In the baking pan, pour the mixture and scatter it into an even layer.

5. Bake until the egg is set, for 12 to 15 minutes.

6. Then leave to cool slightly and cut into squares to eat.

Nutrition information: 235 calories, 15g of fat, 21g of protein, 2.5g of carbohydrates, 0.5g of fiber, 2g of net carbohydrates.

5.2 Recipes for lunch

1. Three Meat & Cheese Sandwich
Servings: 1 Serving

Prep Time: 30 minutes

Cook time: 5 minutes

Ingredients:

- 2 big eggs,

- 1 pinch cream of tartar

- Pinch of salt

- 1 ounce of softened cream cheese

- 1 ounce of ham cut

- 1 ounce of hard salami cut

- 1 ounce of turkey cut

- 2 cheddar cheese slices

Instructions:

1. Preheat the oven to 300 °F for the bread and line a baking sheet with

Parchment.

2. Beat the egg whites with tartar cream and salt until it becomes soft peaks.

3. Whisk the egg yolk and cream cheese until smooth and pale yellow.

4. Gradually mix the yolk batter into the egg whites until smooth and well mixed.

5. Pour the mixture into two even circles onto the baking dish.

6. Bake until solid and slightly browned, for 25 minutes.

7. Make a sandwich by putting the sliced meat and cheese between two bread slices.

8. With cooking oil, grease a skillet and heat over low flame.

9. Keep the sandwich on the skillet and cook until the bottom has browned, then flip and cook until the cheese melts.

Nutrition Information: 610 calories, 48g of fat, 40g of protein, 3g of carbohydrates,

 0.5g of fiber, 2.5g of carbohydrates

2. Kebabs of Beef and Pepper
Servings: 2 Servings

Prep time: 30 minutes

Cook time: 10 minutes

Ingredients:

- 2 teaspoons of olive oil

- 1 1/2 teaspoons of balsamic vinegar

- 2 teaspoons of Dijon mustard

- Salt and pepper

- Beef sirloin, 8 ounces, sliced into 2-inch pieces

- 1 tiny red pepper, chopped into pieces

- 1 tiny green pepper, chopped into pieces

Instructions:

1. In a small dish, mix the olive oil, balsamic vinegar, and Dijon mustard.

2. Season the steak with salt and pepper and then toss in the marinade.

3. Let it marinate for 30 minutes, then slide it with peppers onto skewers.

4. Preheat the grill pan to high flame and use the cooking spray to grease.

5. Cook the kebabs on either side for 2 to 3 minutes until the beef is cooked.

Nutrition Information: 365 calories, 21.5g of fat, 35.5g of protein, 6.5g of carbohydrates, 1.5g of fiber, 5g of net carbohydrates

3. Chicken tenders with Coconut
Servings: 4 Servings

Prep time: 10 minutes

Cook time: 30 minutes

Ingredients:

- 1/4 cup of almond flour

- 2 teaspoons of unsweetened shredded coconut

- 1/2 tablespoons of garlic powder

- 2 pounds of boneless chicken

- Salt and pepper

- 2 big eggs, well whisked,

Instructions:

1. Preheat the oven to 400 ° F and use parchment to cover a baking sheet.

2. In a small bowl, mix the almond flour, coconut, and garlic powder.

3. Season the chicken with salt and pepper, then dip in the beaten eggs.

4. In the almond flour mixture, dredge the chicken tenders, then place them on

the baking sheet.

5. Bake for 25 to 30 minutes, until baked and browned. Serve it hot.

Nutrition Facts: 325 calories, 9.5g of fat, 56.5g of protein, 2g of carbohydrates, 1g

of fiber, 1g net carbohydrates.

4. Ham, Egg & Cheese Sandwich
Servings: 1 Serving:

Prep time: 30 minutes

Cook time: 5 minutes

Ingredients:

- 2 big eggs

- Tartar pinch milk

- Pinch of salt

- 1 ounce of cream cheese, melted

- 1 butter teaspoon

- 3 ounces of ham cut

- 1 cheddar cheese slice

Instructions

1. Preheat the oven to 300 °F for the bread and line a baking sheet with

Parchment.

2. Beat the egg whites with tartar cream and salt until becomes soft peaks.

3. Whisk the egg yolk and cream cheese until smooth and pale yellow.

4. Mix the egg yolk batter into egg whites until smooth and well mixed.

5. Pour the batter into two even circles onto the baking dish.

6. Bake approx. for 25 minutes until it becomes firm and slightly brown.

7. Fry the egg in butter until it's done as per your requirement.

8. On top of one bread circle, place the sliced ham.

9. Cover that with the sliced cheese and the fried egg, then the second circle of bread.

10. Serve immediately or toast it until cheese is melt.

Nutrition information: 530 calories, 40g of fat, 36g of protein, 5.5g of

carbohydrates, 1g of fiber, 4.5g of total carbohydrates.

5.Curried Chicken Soup
Servings: 4 Servings:

Prep time: 10 minutes

Cook time: 20 minutes

Ingredients:

- 2 teaspoons of olive oil

- 4 thighs of boneless chicken (about 12 ounces)

- 1 tiny yellow, chopped onion

- 2 teaspoons of curry powder

- 2 teaspoons of cumin seed powder

- Pinch of cayenne

- 4 cups of cauliflower

- 4 cups of chicken broth

- 1 cup of water

- 2 minced garlic cloves

- 1/2 cup of canned coconut milk

- 2 cups of chopped kale

- Freshly chopped cilantro

Instructions:

1. Chop the chicken into bite-sized pieces and put it aside.

2. Over medium flame, heat 1 tablespoon of oil in a saucepan.

3. Sauté the onions for 4 minutes, then add half the spices to it.

4. Add the cauliflower and sauté further four minutes.

5. Add water and garlic to the broth and boil it.

6. Low the flame and cook for 10 minutes until the cauliflower softens.

7. Remove from the heat and add kale and coconut milk.

8. In a pan, heat the remaining oil and cook the chicken until it turns golden brown.

9. Stir in the remaining spices and cook until the chicken has been done.

10. Mix the chicken with broth and serve it hot, garnished with fresh cilantro.

Nutrition Information: 390 calories, 22 g fat, 34 g protein, 14.5 g carbohydrates,

4.5g fiber, 10 g net carbohydrates.

5.3. Recipes for dinner

1. Baked Lamb Chops with Asparagus
Servings: 4 Servings

Time to prep: 5 minutes

Cook time: 15 minutes

Ingredients:

- 8 bone-in chops of lamb

- Salt and pepper

- 1 tablespoon freshly chopped rosemary

- 1 tablespoon of olive oil

- 1 tablespoon of butter

- 16 asparagus spears, sliced into 2-inch chunks

Instructions:

1. Season the salt and pepper with the lamb and sprinkle the rosemary.

2. Heat oil over medium-high flame in a large skillet.

3. Put the lamb chops and cook until seared, on both sides, for 2 to 3 minutes.

1. Remove the chops from the skillet and keep them aside, then reheat the pan with butter.

5. Add the asparagus to the pan and cover it with a lid.

6. Cook until tender-crisp, 4 to 6 minutes, and serve with the lamb.

Nutrition Information: 380 calories, 18.5g of fat, 48g of protein, 4.5g of

carbohydrates, 2.5g of fiber, 2g of net carbohydrates

2.   Kebabs of Lemon Chicken with Vegetables
Servings: 4 Servings

Prep time: 10 minutes

Cook time: 15 minutes

Ingredients:

- 1 pound of boneless thighs of meat, sliced into cubes

- 1/4 cup of olive oil

- 2 teaspoons lemon juice

- 1 teaspoon of garlic minced

- Salt and pepper

- 1 big yellow onion, diced into 2-inch parts

- 1 big red pepper, sliced into 2-inch parts

- 1 big green pepper, sliced into 2-inch fragments

Instructions:

1. Mix the olive oil, lemon juice, garlic, salt, and pepper with the chicken.

2. With the onion and peppers, slide the chicken onto skewers.

3. Preheat a grill and grease the grates on medium-high flame.

4. Grill the skewers from both sides for 2 to 3 minutes until the chicken is cooked.

Nutrition information: 360 calories, 21g of fat, 34g of protein, 8g of carbohydrates,

2g of fiber, 6g of net carbohydrates.

3. Spicy Chicken Enchilada Casserole
Servings: 6 Servings

Prep Time: Fifteen minutes

Cook time: 1 hour

Ingredients:

- 2 pounds of boneless thighs of meat, sliced

- Salt and pepper

- 3 cups of salsa tomatoes

- 1 1/2 cups cheddar cheese shredded

- 3/4 cup of whipped cream

- 1 cup of diced avocado

- **Instructions:**

1. Preheat the oven to 375 F and grease a tray with a casserole.

2. Season the chicken with pepper and salt and spread it over the plate.

3. Spread the tomato salsa on the chicken and sprinkle the cheeses.

4. Cover the tray tightly with foil, and bake until the chicken is cooked, for 60 minutes.

5. Enjoy sour cream and sliced avocado.

Nutrition Information: 550 calories, 31.5g of fat, 54g of protein, 12g of carbohydrates, 4g of fiber, 8g of net carbohydrates

4. White Cheddar Broccoli Chicken Casserole
Servings: 6 Servings:

Prep Time: 15 minutes

Cook time: 30 minutes

Ingredients:

- 2 teaspoons of olive oil

- 1 pound boneless thighs of meat, chopped

- 1 yellow medium onion, chopped

- 1 garlic clove, minced

- 1 1/2 cups Chicken broth

- Cream cheese 8 ounces, melted

- 1/4 cup of sour cream

- 2 and a half cups of broccoli florets

- 3/4 cup of white cheddar cheese sliced

Instructions:

1. Preheat the oven to 350 F and grease a tray with a casserole.

2. Heat oil over medium-high flame in a large skillet.

3. Add the chicken and cook till golden brown for 2 to 3 minutes.

4. Stir in the garlic and onion, then season with salt and pepper.

5. Sauté for 4 to 5 minutes before the chicken is thoroughly cooked.

6. Mix the chicken broth into the mixture, then add the cream cheese and sour cream.

7. Simmer until it is melted with the cream cheese, then stir in the broccoli.

8. In the casserole bowl, pour the mixture and sprinkle it with cheese.

9. Bake until hot and bubbly, for 25 to 30 minutes.

Nutrition Information: 435 calories, 32g of fat, 29.5g of protein, 6g of

carbohydrates, 1.5g of fiber, 4.5g of net carbohydrates

5. Stuffed Bell Peppers Bacon

Servings: 4 Servings

Prep Time: Fifteen minutes

Cook time: 45 minutes

Ingredients:

- 1 cauliflower, medium head, chopped

- 1 tablespoon of olive oil

- 12 ounces' Italian ground sausage

- 1 tiny yellow, chopped onion

- 1 dried oregano teaspoon

- Salt and pepper

- 4 medium peppers of the bell

Instructions:

1. Preheat the oven to 350°F.

2. Finely chop the cauliflower into rice-like grains in a food processor.

3. Heat the oil over medium heat in a pan, then Cook the cauliflower until tender.

4. Keep the cauliflower rice aside, then reheat the skillet.

5. Add the sausage and fry, also drain the fats once it's done.

6. Stir in the cauliflower with the bacon, mix the cabbage, oregano, salt, and pepper.

7. Slice off the pepper's tops, remove the seeds and pith and pour a little amount of mixture in it.

8. In a baking dish, put the peppers upright, then cover the platter with foil.

9. Bake for 30 minutes, then uncover it and bake for another 15 minutes. Serve it

hot.

Nutrition Information: 355 calories, 23.5g of fat, 19g of protein, 16.5g of carbohydrates, 6g of fiber, 10.5g total carbohydrates

5.4. Keto dessert recipes

1.   Cashew Macadamia Fat Bomb Bars
Servings: 16

Prep Time: 10 minutes

Cook Time: None

Ingredients:

- 1/2 cup of almond butter

- 1/4 cup of unsweetened cocoa powder

- 1/4 cup of erythritol powder

- 2 cups of sliced macadamia nuts

- 1/2 cup of heavy cream

Instructions:

1. In a shallow saucepan over a low fire, melt the almond butter.

2. Whisk in the cocoa powder and sweeten it with erythritol.

3. Stir in the heavy cream and sliced macadamia nuts until well mixed.

4. Pour the mixture into silicone molds and let them cool.

5. Place the molds into the fridge and refrigerate until they harden.

6. Pop out the fat bombs from molds and store them in an airtight jar.

Nutrition Info: 185 calories, 19.5g of fat, 2.5g of protein, 4.5g of carbohydrates, 2.5g

of fiber, 2g of net carbohydrates.

2.   Coconut Truffles from Cocoa
Servings: 12 Servings:

Prep Time: Fifteen minutes

Time for Cook: Zero

Ingredients:

- 1 bottle of coconut butter

- 6 teaspoons of unsweetened ground cocoa

- 2 teaspoons of shredded coconut unsweetened

- 2 teaspoons Instant coffee powder

- Liquid extract of stevia, to taste

- 2 teaspoons of molten coconut oil

Instructions:

1. In the microwave, warm the coconut butter and stir until smooth.

2. Stir in the chocolate, coconut, stevia, and coffee powder.

3. Grease the ice cube tray with molten coconut oil.

4. Spoon the mixture of coconut chocolate into the ice cube tray and pat it flat.

5. Freeze for 4 hours or until firm, then defrost 15 minutes before serving.

Nutrition information: 290 calories, 28g of fat, 3.5g of protein, 11g of

carbohydrates, 8g of fiber, 3g of net carbohydrates.

3.   Chocolate Sun butter
Servings: 16 Servings:

Time to prep: 5 minutes

Time for Cook: Zero

Ingredients:

- 1 cup of coconut oil

- 1 cup of butter of sunflower seed

- 1/2 cup of unsweetened cocoa powder

- 1/4 cup of coconut flour

- Liquid extract of stevia, to taste

Instructions:

1. In a small pan, melt the coconut oil and sunflower seed butter together.

2. Whisk together the coconut flour, ¼ cocoa powder, and

Stevia liquid to taste.

3. Remove from the heat and allow to cool until slightly hardened.

4. Divide it into 16 pieces and roll it into balls and put it in a dish.

5. Coat the fat bombs with remaining cocoa powder and chill.

Nutrition information: 230 calories, 22g of fat, 4g of protein, 8g of carbohydrates,

2g of fiber, 6g of net carbohydrates.

4. Coco-Almond Bomb Bars of Fat
Servings: 12 Servings:

Prep time: 10 minutes

Time for Cook: Zero

Ingredients:

- 1/2 cup of peanut butter

- 1/4 cup of unsweetened cocoa powder

- 1/4 cup of erythritol powder

- 2 cups of toasted almonds, sliced

- 1/2 cup of heavy cream

Instructions:

1. Melt the cocoa butter in a small saucepan over low heat.

2. Whisk in the cocoa powder and sweeten with erythritol.

3. Stir in the chopped almonds and heavy cream until well combined.

4. Pour the mixture into molds of silicone and let them cool.

5. Keep the molds in the fridge and refrigerate until they are hard.

6. Pop out the fat bombs from molds and store them in an airtight jar.

Nutrition Info: 205 calories, 20.5g fat, 4.5g protein, 5g carbs, 3g fiber, 2g

net carbohydrates

5.   Chocolate-Dipped Pecan Fat Bombs
Servings: 16 Servings:

Period for Prep: 10 minutes

Time for Cook: Zero

Ingredients:

- 1 bottle of coconut butter

- 1 cup canned coconut milk

- 1 cup finely chopped pecans

- 1 teaspoon vanilla extract

- Liquid extract of stevia, to taste

- ¼ cup chopped dark chocolate

- ½ teaspoon palm shortening

Instructions:

1. Mix the coconut butter and coconut milk in a small saucepan over low

   heat.

2. When the mixture melted, Stir in the pecans and vanilla, then add sweetener.

3. Remove from flame and chill for 1 to 2 hours until firm.

4. Divide the mixture into 16 pieces and make small balls.

5. Melt the dark chocolate in the microwave with the palm shortening.

6. Dip the balls in the chocolate and place them on a plate

7. Chill until the chocolate is hardened, then serve.

Nutrition Info: 245 calories, 24.5g fat, 3g protein, 9.5g carbs, 5.5g fiber, 4g net carbs

Conclusion

We have reached this juncture and I am so happy that you have selected to take the steps required on this ketogenic voyage. I hope, this book and its contents, will be able to give you step by step actionable value, for your efforts toward nutritional ketosis. More significantly, I hope that the book has also given you the self-confidence booster and has built up your promise to stay on the diet.

One of the main keys to any successful diet or lifestyle change has always been the choice of correct nutrients that fit in with the doctrines of the diet. Overall, eating moderate protein, rich fat, and low carbs might have an enormous influence on your health – dropping your body weight, cholesterol, blood sugar, and raising your mood levels and energy.

A ketogenic diet can be tough to fathom at the start but isn't as inflexible as it's made out to be. The alteration can be a little bit tough, but the increasing popularity of the clean eating program makes it easier and easier to find accessible low-carb foods. In the end, I would claim that this book is devoted to anyone who still unnecessarily trusts in traditional dietary advice, particularly if it has never helped them lose weight or get healthier and most definitely made things drastically worse.

Thanks a million, stay healthy and happy!

KETO FOR WOMEN AFTER 50

The Ultimate Ketogenic Diet Step by Step To Learn How to Easily Lose Weight for Woman and Feel Younger

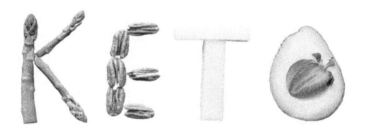

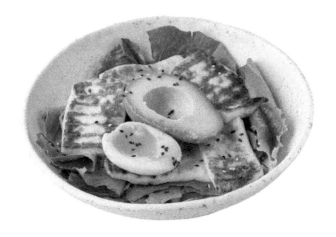

Introduction

The increasing age, deterioration in physiological function, metabolic dysfunction, poor immunity makes a person vulnerable to a number of chronic diseases. So, you now have to start worrying about your health if you're over 50. Picture what life would be like, when a simple diet change could almost immediately make you look years younger.

The keto diet, particularly for weight loss, is very common worldwide because of its many advantages. You will just be capable of taking your body to a whole new level when you adopt this diet and regain the youthful nature also after 50 years of age.

Ketogenic diets and Atkins allow followers to eliminate carbohydrates from their foods. Thus, while the Atkins diet lowers the calories steadily over time, Keto sets strict limits on carbohydrates and protein. The carbohydrate system is depleted by this eating practice, forcing it to consume fat and help create an extra supply of energy called ketones. A conventional ketogenic diet restricts carbohydrates to less than 10% of calories and 20% of protein, while the rest is fat.

Losing weight is only the beginning. Research has demonstrated a stabilized emotional state. It enhances energy rates. Regulate your blood sugar. It lowers blood pressure, boosts potassium, and many have personally seen the outcomes in their lives.

In addition to traditional therapies, including chemotherapy for many other cancers that affect women, including glioblastoma multiforme, aggressive cancer that affects the brain, the ketogenic diet so far has shown potential results when used as a treatment.

Today, life is characterized by packaged and refined food containing tons of sugar, low energy, anxiety, and depression. Many people are frightened by Keto. They may not have a decent amount of money to eat these. Or perhaps they are afraid of losing their favorite meal.

The insights and recipes included in this guide can get you started on your journey to a healthy, fitter body, even though you suffer from age-related ailments or obesity over the age of 50 years.

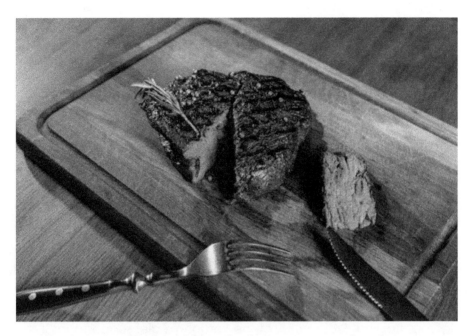

Looking to lose weight and keep in shape as you get on in years can be very challenging, especially when you're a woman. Your body is not as supple as it used to be once, and the body's metabolism has been slowed down to a great extent. But it doesn't need to be like that. There's a way to accelerate one's metabolism and be the healthiest and fittest version one has ever been, and you will get to know about that all in the Keto Diet.

1.1 How does body routine requirements modify once the 50-year Rubicon is reached?

You often come across people who have a high metabolism rate. Such people, despite consuming large quantities of food are slim. That quick metabolism very effectively processes that food. Now, these people do not only have a metabolism that is genetically fast, but they may also be younger and may also have more lean muscle mass, which will more effectively burn the calories. They may also be individuals who consume a lot of calories, but they will be balanced calories such as proteins, fats, or carbohydrates.

1.2 Simple comprehension of keto diet mechanism

The concept of weight loss in the ketogenic diet is that alternative fuel ketones are produced from the stored fat if one deprives the body of glucose (thus "keto" genic) — the essential energy source for all body cells obtained from eating fatty foods. The brain's routine requirement of glucose is about 120 g a day, most often in constant supply, so glucose could not really be processed in there. The body first eliminates the stored glucose from the liver by fasting, even though when too little carbohydrate is consumed, and breaks down the muscle momentarily to eliminate glucose. As this occurs for 3- 4 days before the stored glucose becomes completely depleted, hormone blood levels are named insulin to drop. The body begins using fat as a primary energy source. The liver makes ketone bodies out of fat, which can be used when there is no glucose available.

The term is called Ketosis, when the ketone bodies start to gather in one's body. When the ketone bodies start to gather in one's body, the term is called Ketosis. Normally, young individuals experience mild Ketosis through fasting periods (e.g., nighttime sleeping) and very rigorous training. Proponents of the ketogenic diet suggest that if the diet is followed very carefully, blood levels of ketones will not reach a harmful amount ('ketoacidosis') because the brain will use ketones for food, and healthy young people can produce adequate insulin to prevent the formation of excessive ketones. How rapidly Ketosis occurs and the number of ketone bodies circulating in the blood varies from person to person, based on factors such as body fat percentage and metabolic rest rate.

1.3 What are the relevant considerations for women over the age of 50

Over the increasing age, the metabolic rate starts to slow down. You appear to conserve more calories with age. The metabolic rate could also be modified by the food types you consume, how much you eat certain foods, and your physical activity level. If women over 50 years of age person don't really reduce their calorie intake as they tend to age, and their physical activity does not increase, they may begin to gain weight.

Temptation, desires, social stigma, physical exhaustion, and mental grogginess ("keto fog") may cause those uncertain of what lies ahead to suddenly quit and return to their former foods over the first few weeks.

During those inaugural weeks, when the body is totally shifting its primary energy source from carbs to fats, here are a few ways to stay on track.

1. Regularly update the necessities

When adopting the keto lifestyle, choose to make sure you get all the nutrients you really need while your general health is in tip-top condition. Just because you shift to Keto, this doesn't really mean you're going to start eating awful stodgy items. Do not follow those websites that are boring. Keto could be fun-loving. This isn't about consuming trash. It's about offering only what your body needs, and that also includes your taste buds.

2. Keto-friendly holiday feast with mates

What's worse than being that guy on the table in a restaurant who can't eat anything? Before heading out, prepare your homework. Check out the popular suggested restaurants to find out if there is anything on the menu that suits you. Browse the restaurants' online menus or pick up a telephone to reach them. It's fantastic to have a dream restaurant. Find it out and visit these for your pleasure with your mates and enjoy a perfect holiday keto feast.

3. Staying hydrated while working out a bit more

Regular exercise helps remove the glycogen in one's system, helping you to more quickly burn the calories on Keto. It'll take a couple of days for your body to adapt to the Keto diet and begin to achieve the results you're looking for in weight loss. So, don't be hard on yourself. Slow and gradual workouts do the trick.

It's always necessary to remain hydrated when eating the right stuff. Get a refillable water bottle. Take it with you and fill it, striving for at least 2 liters of water a day. Keeping healthful with stress-free exercises, helps the body to pass through Ketosis and take away more fat while being beneficial for the whole body, soul, and mind.

4. Don't obsess & get ready to feel smart

You shouldn't really be worrying 24 hours a day about what next to eat on Keto. Yes, particularly at first, the diet seems intense, but it does not have to be the entire focus of your day. When you strike the sweet spot of energy, do this on work or hobbies and embrace it. It is believed that Ketosis shakes out brain fog. If that sounds right to you, this could be a perfect time to start a new project at work that needs intense focus.

5. Prepare yourself for compliments.

It's good and fun to say that you're on Keto and have lost weight, you're going to be praised by people in your life, and that's motivating. You can lose five pounds and then, for no reason at all, regain it. It's not you—it's a natural adaptation of your body. Shrug it off and continue to move on. Eating a wide range of healthy foods on Keto keeps your levels of nutrients high and avoids boredom to boot.

1.5 How to minimize common misconceptions
1. Nervous about eating too much fat

When people start Keto, they sometimes do not consume adequate fat because our culture has been conditioned to assume that fats can make you fat. Since you're reducing keto carb intake, it's important to replace those calories with fat calories. If you just don't have enough calories, your hormonal function and metabolism can be affected in the long term. All fats really aren't considered equal, and since fats are the basis of the ketogenic diet, it is important that the right sources of fat are eaten.

2. There Isn't enough Sodium Intake

When one's body runs on ketones for energy, sodium is released alongside the water. You may fall prey to the dreaded flu, which is the primary cause for not substituting your electrolytes if you do not switch your sodium on Keto. To stop this, boost sodium intake by salting each meal, introducing pink Himalayan sea salt to your water and drinking it during the day, and also consuming broth from bouillon cubes, boost your sodium intake.

3. Too much obsession with the scale

While the ketogenic diet is recognized for its immense weight loss benefits, an accurate reading is not always shown on the scale. You will experience water weight loss over the first few days after starting Keto for the first time. But it will hold some water until the body has adjusted to this new type of diet. Several times a day, testing your weight would just prevent you from holding on to the ketogenic diet because weights normally fluctuate.

1.6 Can this ketogenic diet pose any danger to women?

Interestingly, although some research suggests that some risk factors for heart disease, including LDL (bad) cholesterol, may be increased by the ketogenic diet, however other studies have shown that the diet may support heart health.

Whether you should follow the keto diet relies on many factors. It is important to weigh the positive and negative aspects of the diet, as well as its suitability, based on your current state of health before you begin any major dietary changes.

For instance, for a woman with obesity, diabetes, or who is unable to lose weight or control her blood sugar by using dietary changes, the ketogenic diet may be an acceptable alternative. On the other hand, the diet is not safe for pregnant or breastfeeding women.

While some women may find success in adopting a ketogenic dietary pattern, it is probably more effective for the majority of women to pursue a less restrictive, healthy diet that can be maintained for life

Rely on your health and nutritional requirements, and it's often recommended to follow a dietary pattern that is rich in whole, nutritionally sound foods that can be preserved for life

1.7 Certain benefits of Keto for fitness

Surveys have shown that diet can benefit a large range of different health conditions.

- Cancer: The diet is currently being considered as an alternative cancer treatment, as it could help delay the growth of tumors.

- Ovarian polycystic syndrome: Insulin levels may also be lowered by a ketogenic diet, which can play a vital role in polycystic ovary syndrome.

- Alzheimer's disease: The keto diet will help relieve Alzheimer's disease symptoms and delay its development.

- Brain injuries: Some findings indicate that this diet can improve the results of brain trauma injuries.

- Epilepsy: Current study has also shown that a ketogenic diet in epileptic children can cause substantial reductions in seizures.

Chapter 2: Breakfast Recipes

1. Classic bacon and eggs

Cook time: 10 mins, Servings: 4, Difficulty: easy

Ingredients

- Eggs 8
- Sliced bacon 9.oz
- Cherry tomatoes (optional)
- Thyme (Fresh)

Instructions

1. On medium heat, fry the bacon in a saucepan until it gets crispy. Hold it aside on a plate. The rendered fat is to be left in the pan.

2. The same pan is used for frying the eggs. Pan is placed over medium heat, and eggs are cracked into the bacon grease. To

prevent splattering of hot grease, you can also break them into a measuring cup and then carefully pour them into the pan.

3. Cook the eggs the way you prefer them. Let the eggs fry on one side for a sunny side up and cover the pan with a lid to ensure they are fried on top. Continue cooking for another 1 minute and then flip the eggs. Cherry tomatoes are cut in half and simultaneously fried.

4. Add pepper and salt to taste.

Nutrition

Kcal: 377, fat 32 g, Protein 20 g, net carbs one g.

2. Spinach and feta breakfast scramble

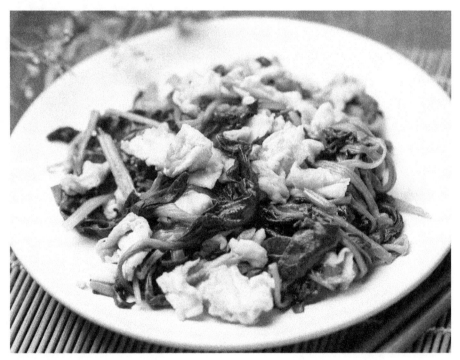

Cook time: 5-10 mins, Servings: 2, Difficulty: easy

Ingredients

- Large eggs 4
- Whipping cream2 tbsp. (heavy)
- Butter 2 tbsps.

- Baby spinach fresh 4 oz.
- Clove of garlic (minced) 1
- Black pepper (salt and ground)
- Crumbled feta cheese 1½ oz. Feta
- Bacon 4 oz.

Instructions

1. We whisk the eggs and cream together in a medium bowl until well blended.

2. Over medium-low heat, the large skillet is heated, and then butter is added. Stir the spinach and garlic and let the butter melt. Cook till the spinach is wilted. Use salt and pepper to sprinkle.

3. The egg mixture is poured into the skillet and cooked until it starts to set around the edges. Gently lift the batter with the help of a rubber spatula from the edge of the pan towards the center. Continue to turn and lift until the eggs are set according to your taste.

4. Take off the pan from the stove and sprinkle feta cheese. Add a few fried bacon slices depending on your liking and serve quickly.

Nutrition

Kcal: 348, fat 30 g, Protein 16 g, net carbs 3 g

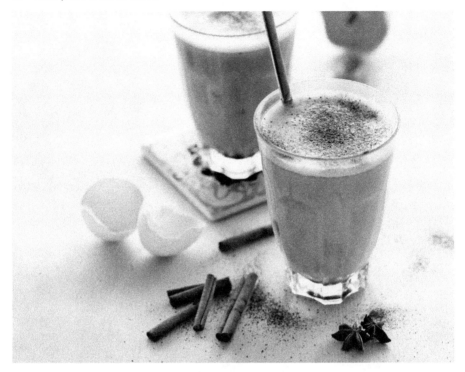

Cook time: 5 mins, Servings: 2, Difficulty: easy

Ingredients

- Eggs 2
- Coconut oil 2 tbsps.
- Cups of coffee 1 1/2
- Extract of vanilla1 pinch
- Pumpkin pie spice(ground ginger) 1 tsp

Instructions

1. Blend in a blender with all the ingredients. You have to be quick so that the eggs do not cook in the boiling water. Immediately drink.

Nutrition

Kcal 193, fat 18 g, Protein 6 g, net carbs 1 g

4. Avocado eggs served with bacon sails

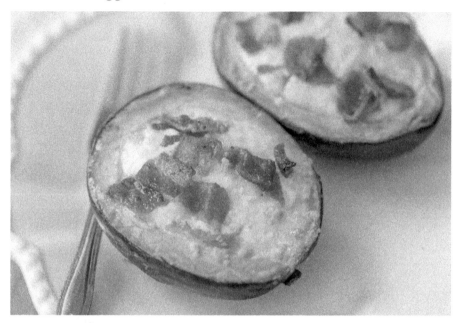

Cook time: 20 mins, Servings 4, Difficulty: easy

Ingredients

- Bacon2½ oz.
- Eggs of large size 2
- Avocado½ (3½ oz.)
- olive oil1 tsp
- Pepper and salt

Instructions

2. Preheat oven to 180°C (350°F). With the help of parchment paper/ foil, line a rimmed baking sheet. Lay the strips of bacon over baking sheet and set them aside.

3. In a saucepan, place the eggs at least 1 inch more than the eggs with cold water. Cover & bring to a slight boil over a high flame. Once the eggs are boiled, take off the pan from the burner and let remaining of the eggs for 15 minutes afterward,

covered in the pan. Put eggs to an ice-cold water bowl, using a slotted spoon for about 5-10 minutes, or put them inside colander. Place them under chilled water until they are fully cooled. Peel them, and then set them aside.

4.   Inside the middle oven rack, arrange the baking sheet and cook bacon for a duration of 10-20 minutes (time varies with thickness), or till it appears crispy. Dry out bacon over paper towels. When it gets cold, shape the sails.

5.   Lengthwise, slice the eggs and scoop the yolks out. In a small bowl, put olive oil, yolks and avocado. The fork is used to mash them until combined. It is then seasoned with salt and pepper to taste.

6.   To assemble, spoon out mixture of avocado yolk generously to the egg whites, and arrange bacon sails in the middle of the mixed blend. Cherish and enjoy the unbeatable taste.

Nutrition

Kcal 152, fat 14 g, Protein 6 g, net carbs 1 g

5.   Chocolate Keto Protein Shake

Cook time: 5 mins, Servings: 1, Difficulty: easy.

Ingredients

- Almond milk 3/4 c
- Ice1/2 c
- Butter with almonds2 tbsps.
- Cocoa powder (unsweetened) 2 tbsps.
- A sugar substitute for taste such as Swerve 2 - 3 tbsps.
- Seeds of chia can use more for serving1 tbsps.
- Seeds of hemp could use more for serving2 tbsp.
- Vanilla extract (pure form) 1/2 tbsp.
- Pinch kosher salt

Instructions

1. Combine all the blender ingredients and blend until fluffy. Pour chia and hemp seeds for garnishing.

Nutrition

Kcal 440, fat 31.2g g, protein 15.6 g, net carbs 8.2 g

6. Bunless Bacon, Egg & Cheese

Cook time: 10 mins, Servings: 1, Difficulty: easy

Ingredients

- Big eggs2
- Water2 tbsp.
- Avocado, finely mashed1/2
- Cooked slice of bacon, halved 1
- Shredded cheddar1/4 c

Instructions

2. Take two Mason jar lids with centers removed in a medium non-stick pan. The entire pan is to be sprayed with cooking spray and then placed over medium heat. Try to crack the eggs into the centers of the lids and whisk gently to crack the yolk with a fork.

3. Cover the pan by pouring water around the lids. Steam the eggs until the whites are cooked, like for about 3 minutes. Remove the lid. Spread the cheddar on one egg and allow it to cook for about 1 minute so that cheese melts.

4. Turn the side of egg bun onto a tray while not having cheese. Place the avocado and bacon on top. Place the egg bun topped with cheese on top, cheese side down.

Nutrition

Kcal 460, fat 13 g, Protein 27 g, net carbs 8.4 g

7. Avocado Egg Boats

Cook time: 10 mins, Servings: 4, Difficulty: easy

Ingredients

- Avocados (ripe), pitted, and halved2.

- Big eggs4
- Kosher salt
- Ground black pepper (fresh)
- Sliced bacon3
- Fresh chopped chives(garnishing)

Instructions

1. Preheat the oven to 350 degrees. From each half of the avocado, scoop about one tablespoon of avocado. Reserve remaining for another time or discard.

2. In a baking dish, put the hollowed avocados and then crack one egg at a time into the pan. With the help of a spoon, pass yolk to avocado half, using a spoon, and spoon in egg white as you can manage and try not to spill over.

3. Bake for about 20 to 25 minutes while seasoning it with salt and pepper until the whites of egg settle down and the yolks are no runnier. (If avocados start to get brown, cover with the foil.)

4. In a bowl over medium flame, cook the bacon for about 8 minutes until it becomes crispy, and then shift it to a plate lined with paper towel. Chop it.

5. When serving, avocados are to be topped with bacon and chives.

Nutrition

Kcal 220, fat 4 g, Protein 6 g, net carbs 7.3 g

8. Loaded Cauliflower Breakfast Bake

Cook time: 15 mins, Servings: 6, Difficulty: easy

Ingredients

- Big cauliflower head1
- Slices of bacon, chopped 8
- Eggs 10
- Whole milk 1 c

- Minced cloves of garlic 2
- Paprika2 tsp
- Kosher salt
- Black pepper
- Crushed cheddar2 c
- Thin sliced green onions, plus more for garnish 2
- Hot sauce to serve

Instructions

1. An oven is preheated to 350 centigrade. On a box grater, grate the head of cauliflower and shift it to a large baking dish.

2. Smoke bacon for about 8 minutes. Inside large skillet medium heat until it becomes crispy. To drain the fat, pass it to a paper towel-lined tray.

3. Whisk the milk, eggs, garlic, and paprika together into a large bowl. Season it with salt and pepper and salt.

4. The cauliflower is topped with cooked bacon, green onions, and cheddar cheese and poured over the egg mixture.

5. This should be baked for 35 to 40 minutes until the eggs are firm and the top gets golden brown in color.

6. It is then garnished with hot sauce and some more green onions.

7. Ready to be served.

Nutrition

Kcal 390, fat 27 g, Protein 28 g, net carbs 6.2 g

9. Spinach Tomato Frittata - Keto

Cook time: 10 mins, Servings: 8, Difficulty: easy

Ingredients

- Big eggs 8
- A cup of spinach 3
- A cup of cherry tomatoes 2

- Bacon chopped slices 8

- Garlic powder 1 tsp

- A cup of cheese (shredded) 1

- Salt

- Black pepper

Instructions

1. First, the oven is preheated to 350 °. A 9-10' deep pie dish is buttered, which is then set aside.

2. Put the bacon on a 12-inch non-stick skillet and cook it on medium-high heat for about 6 to 10 minutes by tossing it frequently until it gets crispy and brown in color.

3. To dry out the bacon, shift it to a plate lined with multiple layers of paper towels. Leave about one tablespoon of bacon fat into the drain of the skillet and reserve or discard excess.

4. Again, put the skillet on a medium-high flame; add on the spinach and tomatoes. Sauté this for about 15 seconds. Move the spinach along with bacon to a plate.

5. Mix well the eggs and garlic powder in a bowl, whisk them until well blended. Now season it with salt and pepper according to taste.

6. Toss the mixture so that ingredients distribute well by adding cooked bacon, spinach, and mozzarella cheese together. Pour this on a dish of the prepared pie.

7. For about 30 – 35 mins, bake it till it settles. It is almost done when a knife inserted in the middle comes out clean. Split into wedges and serve it warm to eat.

Nutrition

Kcal 134, fat 26 g, protein 10 g, net carbs 6 g

1. The keto bread

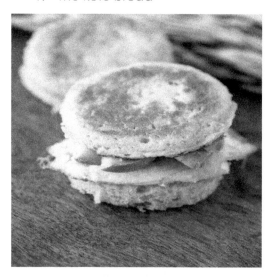

Cook time: 1 hr. +10 mins, Servings: 6, Difficulty: medium

Ingredients

- A cup of ground psyllium husk powder 1/3
- Cups of almond flour 1 ¼
- Baking powder 2 tsp
- Sea salt 1 tsp
- A cup of water 1
- Cider vinegar 2 tsp
- Egg whites 3
- Sesame seeds 2 tbsp.

Instructions

1. The oven is preheated to 175°C (350°F).
2. In a large mixing bowl, the dry ingredients are mixed. Boil the water.
3. To the dry ingredients, add on vinegar and egg whites, and mix them well. Boiling water is added while beating for

approximately 30 seconds with a hand mixer. Don't mix the dough too much; the consistency should be similar to Play-Doh.

4. By applying a little olive oil, moisten the hands. Make six separate rolls from the dough. Place it on a baking sheet that is greased. Top it with sesame seeds (optional).

5. Bake in the oven for 50-60 minutes on the lower rack, based on the bread rolls' size. For confirming, tap the bottom of the bun. A hollow sound could be sensed while tapping the bread, which is an indication that bread is done and is ready to be served.

6. Serve it with butter and toppings depending upon choice.

Nutrition

Kcal 165, fat 12g, Protein 6 g, net carbs 2 g

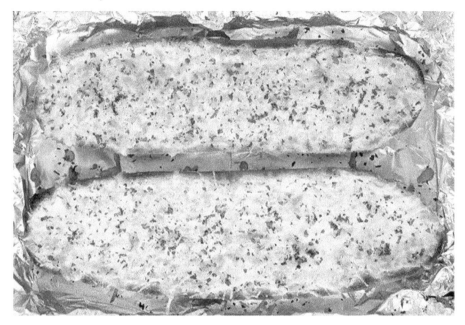

Cook time: 25 mins, Servings: 10, Difficulty: medium

Ingredients

- Bread Base
- Almond flour (Well bee's)1 1/4 C
- Coconut flour 1 T
- Beaten egg whites 3
- Olive oil /avocado oil 2 T
- Lukewarm water 1/4 C
- Yeast (granular form) 1 tsp.
- Coconut sugar (honey)1 tsp
- Mozzarella cheese (shredded) 1/2 C
- Salt 1/4 tsp
- Baking powder 2 tsp.
- Garlic powder 1/4 tsp.

- Xanthan gum (optional) 1/2 tsp.

Topping

- A cup of mozzarella cheese(shredded) 1
- Melted butter 2 T
- Garlic powder 1/4 tsp.
- Salt 1/4 tsp.
- Italian seasoning 1/2 tsp.

Instructions

1. Preheat the oven to 400°C.
2. Mix coconut flour, almond, salt, baking powder, garlic powder, and xanthan gum together in a large cup. Stir them all well.
3. Add warm water and sugar to a shallow bowl. Stir them to dissolve, and then add yeast. Leave it aside for a few mins.
4. With the help of a rubber spatula, apply olive oil and yeast-water mixture to the flour mixture, and then stir it with the help of a rubber spatula. Add on beaten eggs while mixing.
5. Mozzarella shreds 1/2 Care added to the mixture with gentle mixing using a spatula until the cheese is well combined and pleasant dough is formed.
6. Grease a 9-9 square cake pan or large sheet of cookies. Pour the batter onto a cookie sheet or cake pan. On the cookie sheet, loosely shape the dough into a rectangle or square.
7. Bake at about 400 degrees, approximately for 15-17 mins or until the crust sides turn golden brown. Now remove it and top.
8. Just mix the butter, garlic powder, and salt in a tiny bowl and brush over the base of the garlic bread. Make sure the butter gets over every inch.
9. Place the shredded mozzarella cheese on top of the bread, and then sprinkle it with Italian seasoning.
10. Bake it for 10 minutes at 400 degrees, or till the cheese melts. Turn on the broiler for the final 3 minutes to brown the cheese.

11. Take away the bread from the oven and allow it to stand before serving for 5-10 minutes.

Nutrition

Kcal 175, fat 16g, Protein 8 g, net carbs 4 g

3. Almond Buns

Cook time: 15 mins, Servings: 3, Difficulty: easy

Ingredients

- Cups of Bob's Red Mill Almond Flour ¾ cup
- Big Eggs 2
- Unsalted Butter5 Tbsp.
- Splenda (optional)1.5 tsp
- Baking Powder1.5 tsp

Instructions

1. Put the dry ingredients in a bowl and blend.
2. Whisk the eggs together.
3. Melt the butter, blend and whisk in the mixture.
4. Divide the mixture into six sections equally in a Muffin Top tray.
5. Bake it in an oven at 350 degrees for 12–17 minutes.
6. Just allow it cool on a wire rack.

Nutrition

Kcal 373, fat 35g, protein 12 g, net carbs 7.2 g

4. Keto fathead pizza

Cook time: 20 mins, Servings: 8 slices, Difficulty: easy

Ingredients

- A cup of shredded Mozzarella cheese 2 cups
- Cream cheese 2 tbsp.
- Almond Flour 1 cup
- Large egg 1

- Baking powder 1 tsp

- Italian seasoning(optional) 1 tsp

- Garlic powder (optional) 1 tsp

- Toppings

- Fresh mozzarella/ parmesan.

- Pepperoni, turkey.

- Jalapeno/pepper/olives/ spinach.

- Sugar-free tomato sauce/ blue cheese, and buffalo.

- Crushed Red Peppers

Instructions

1. An oven is preheated to 450F.

2. Add cream cheese and mozzarella to a sizeable bowl and microwave them for 45 seconds.

3. After removing from the microwave, add in the egg, garlic, almond flour, baking powder, and Italian seasoning. Mix until well blended, with a spoon.

4. The dough is shifted onto a large piece of parchment paper while covering it with another piece of paper. Flatten the dough to around 1/4 "thick using a rolling pin. Remove the parchment paper and shape it with your hands if necessary.

5. Shift the pizza on a baking sheet or pizza stone over the parchment paper and bake it for 10 minutes.

6. While keeping the oven on, remove the pizza. Serve with all of your favorite sauces and toppings.

7. Bake pizza for another 5-8 minutes or until the cheese is bubbly.

Nutrition

Kcal 249, fat 19g, Protein 14g, net carbs 6.8 g

5. Keto pizza

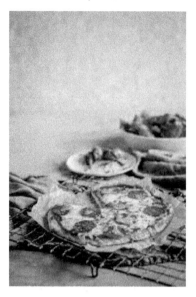

Cook time: 25 mins, Servings: 2 slices, Difficulty: medium

Ingredients

- Crust
- Eggs 4
- Mozzarella cheese (shredded) 1½ cups
- Topping
- Tomato sauce (unsweetened) 3 tbsp.
- Oregano(dried) 1 tsp
- Provolone shredded cheese1¼ cups
- Pepperoni 1½ oz.
- Olives (optional)

For serving

- Leafy greens 1 cup
- A cup of olive oil¼
- Salt
- Black pepper (grounded)

Instructions

1. Preheat the oven to 200 centigrade.

2. Begin by forming the crust. Crack the eggs and add the shredded cheese to a medium-sized dish. Stir it well so that it mixes properly.

3. The baking sheet is lined with parchment paper for spreading the cheese and egg batter. It can be formed in any shape, either form two round circles or just make one big rectangular pizza. Bake for 15 minutes in the oven until the crust of the pizza turns golden. Remove and leave for a minute or two to cool.

4. Raise the temperature of the oven is to 225°C (450°F).

5. Spread the tomato sauce on the crust and top it with sprinkled oregano, some more cheese, pepperoni, and olives on top.

6. Bake it for a time of about 5-10 minutes or until the brown color of the pizza has turned golden.

7. Balance and serve it with a fresh salad.

Nutrition

Kcal 1024, fat 86g, Protein 56g, net carbs 6 g

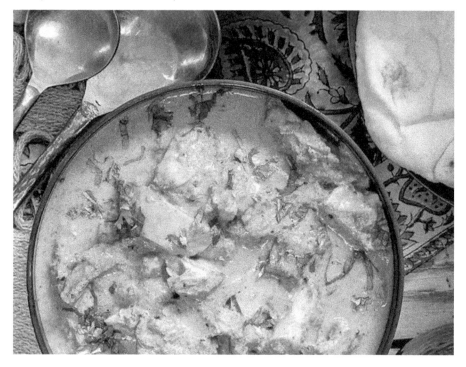

1. Low-carb butter chicken salad

Cook time: 20-25 mins, Servings: 4, Difficulty: easy.

Ingredients

- A cup of Greek yogurt ¾
- Tandoori paste 2½ tbsp.
- Vegetable oil 1 tbsp.
- Garam masala 2½tsp.
- Lily dale Free Range Thigh of Chicken 8
- Red onion, thin slices 1
- Juice of lemon 1

- Caster sugar ¼ tsp.

- Lebanese cucumber, sliced in round shape 1

- Tomatoes small truss halved 250g

- Green chilies (sliced) 2

- Curry leaves chopped 2 tbsp. (optional)

- A big bunch of coriander leaves 1

- A cup of chopped roasted cashews⅓ cup

Instructions

1. In a baking dish, mix 1/4 cup (70g) yogurt, 1 1/2 tbsp. tandoori paste, 1 tbsp. Olive oil and 2 tsp. garam masala, and set it aside.

2. Place two thighs of chicken on a cutting board. To make three separate skewers, pass three skewers through the thighs, and then cut them parallel to the middle skewer. To make 12 skewers, repeat the step. Marinade the skewers to toss until fully covered, using your fingertips. Take at least 30 minutes.

3. Preheat the oven grill and set a shelf in the oven in a lower position. Cover a second baking dish with foil, narrower than the length of the skewers. Place skewers over the prepared dish so that the chicken settles above the dish's surface. Grill it for 10 minutes till slightly charred. Turn the side and grill for an additional 5-10 minutes.

4. In the meantime, in a cup, combine the onion, lemon juice, 1 tsp. Salt, sugar, and the rest of 1/2 tsp. garam masala and shake to blend. Set aside until necessary. Place the cucumber, chili, curry leaves and cilantro in a bowl and set aside until appropriate.

5. Combine in a bowl the remaining 1/2 cup of yogurt and 1 tbsp. All of them are combined to create a swirl effect with a spoon. For cucumber salad, drained pickled onion is added and tossed until well blended. Assemble it on serving plates. Sprinkle over some of the cooking juices. Then add skewers to the dishes. Scatter with cashews and chili leftovers to serve.

Nutrition

Kcal 122, fat 8.7g, protein 10.2g, net carbs 2.6 g

2. Yogurt and lime grilled chicken

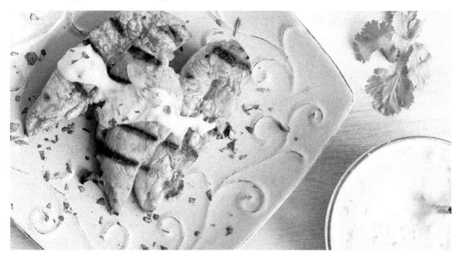

Cook time: 40 mins, Servings: 4, Difficulty: capable.

Ingredient

- Lily dale Free Range Whole Chicken 1.6kg

- A cup of ras el hanout (Moroccan spice) quarter of cup

- Greek-style yoghurt(thick) 1 cup

- Juice of lemon 1

- Virgin olive oil 2 tbsp.

- Lime wedges

Instructions

1. Take breast and leg, slice two shallow slits, and then sprinkle salt flakes all over the chicken.

2. In a big bowl, mix yogurt, ras el hanout, lemon juice, and 1 tsp of salt. Put the chicken and then turn it well to coat. To marinate, chill for a minimum of 2 hours or let it stay overnight.

3. Preheat on a medium-high pan with chargrill and oven it to 180 degrees Celsius. Now pick out the chicken from the fridge 30 minutes before cooking. Take out the chicken from the marinade, allowing the excess to slip away. Glaze with oil and

cook for 5 minutes until it turns golden. Turn and cook, or until golden, for another 5 minutes. Shift it to a baking tray by doing the breast side up and then roast in the oven for 30-40 minutes till the juices start appearing clear when the thigh is pierced with a skewer. In the meantime, close the barbecue hood and reduce the heat to a medium amount. Cook it for about 30-40 minutes. Let it rest for 10 minutes while loosely covered with foil

4. The grilled chicken is then seasoned with salt and served with lime.

Nutrition

Kcal 134, fat 9.4g, protein 10g, net carbs 0.8 g

3. Simple keto meatballs

Cook time: 20 mins, Servings: 1, Difficulty: easy

Ingredients

- Beef (grounded) 1 lb.
- Eggs 1
- A cup of grated parmesan half cup
- A cup of shredded mozzarella half cup
- Garlic (minced) 1 tbsp.
- Blackpepper1 tsp.
- Salt1/2 tsp.
- Perfect keto unflavored whey protein (optional)1 scoop

Instructions

1. Firstly, line the baking sheet with parchment paper by preheating the oven to 400 degrees.
2. Add all the ingredients to a bowl and mix them with the help of your hands and knead until everything is nicely incorporated.
3. Take the mixture and make meatballs of the same size and position them on the prepared baking sheet.
4. Bake it for 18-20 minutes, then.

5. Allow it to cool

6. Serve warm.

Nutrition

Kcal 153, fat 10.9g, protein 12.2g,net carbs 0.7 g

4. Creamy Tuscan garlic butter shrimp

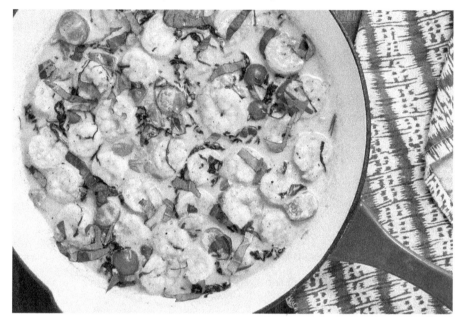

Cook time: 15 mins, Servings: 6, Difficulty: easy

Ingredients

- Butter 2 tbsp.
- Tail-off white medium-sized shrimp (cooked) 2 pounds
- Onion, (small and diced)¼
- Red bell pepper(diced/ chopped) 1
- Cloves garlic(minced) 4-6
- Canned full-fat coconut milk (one/ 13.5 ounce)
- Spinach /kale 2 cups
- Grated parmesan cheese(one/ 5-ounce container)
- Perfect keto unflavouredcollagen3 scoops

- Sea salt 1 tsp
- Black pepper 1 tsp
- Italian seasoning 1 tbsp

Instructions

1. Add on the red bell pepper, shrimp, butter, onion, and minced garlic to large stainless steel over medium-high heat, stir it to combine, and cook until the onions appear translucent in color for around 6-8 minutes.

2. Add coconut milk / heavy cream, sea salt, spinach, pepper, parmesan cheese, and seasoning. Stir them all to mix and bring to a boil.

3. Turn down the heat to medium-low and leave for 15 minutes to simmer.

4. Top it with finely chopped parsley over cauliflower rice or steamed broccoli.

Nutrition

Kcal 334, fat 15.8g, Protein 27.25g, net carbs4 g

5. Keto creamy garlic lemon zucchini pasta

Cook time: 10 mins, Servings: 2, Difficulty: easy

Ingredients

- Zucchini noodles two large
- Olive oil 2tbsp
- Lemon 1 (zest reserved + 1/3 cup of fresh lemon juice)
- Clove of garlic finely minced four cloves.
- Salt½tsp
- Black pepper¼tp
- Cream cup ¼
- Fresh basil/ parsley (a handful of roughly chopped)

Instructions

1. In a large saucepan set over medium heat, add olive oil.

2. Continue cooking by adding garlic for 30 seconds until you could smell the aroma.

3. In the pan, add on with the lemon juice and zest along with salt, pepper, and heavy cream. Cook for 8-10 minutes to minimize the sauce. Adjust the seasoning according to taste. Turn the heat off.

4. Now add on zucchini noodles in it, and then toss in the sauce.

5. Serve it with parmesan chicken or mini meatloaves as an aside. Use herbs for garnishing. Enjoy the meal.

Nutrition

Kcal 283, fat 25g, Protein 4g, net carbs 12 g

6. Keto crescent rolls

Cook time: 30 mins, Servings: 8, Difficulty: medium

Ingredients

Mozzarella cheese4 oz

- Cream cheese(shredded) 2 oz

- Egg 1

- Almond flour cup 1 cup

- Coconut flour cup ¼ cup

- Monk fruit 1tbsp

- Baking powder 1 tsp

- Salt¼ tsp

Instructions

1. In a heat-proof container, add mozzarella and cream cheese. Microwave at intervals of 30 seconds until completely melted.

2. Now whisk the egg and pour into the mixture of cheese.

3. Then add the monk fruit, almond flour, coconut flour, baking powder, and salt to a separate bowl. Whisk in order to combine.

4. Blend wet and dry ingredients together with the spoon.

5. Knead and shape the dough into a small ball. Enroll in a wrap of plastic and cool for 20-30 minutes.

6. An oven is now preheated to 350 °F. Parchment paper is used to line a baking pan.

7. The dough is now taken out of the refrigerator, and the plastic is removed. Press the dough into a rectangular shape using a rolling pin.

8. Shape into a triangle (large end to small end). Roll them to create the classic "crescent roll."

9. Bake them for 20- 25 minutes until they get the golden brown.

Nutrition

Kcal 147, fat 11g, Protein 8g, net carbs 12 g

7. Keto parmesan chicken

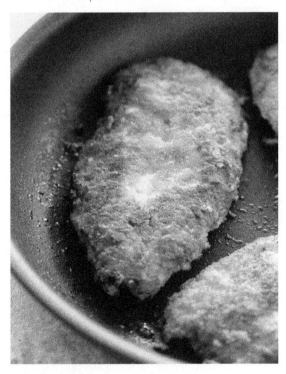

Cook time: 30 mins, Servings: 4, Difficulty: medium.

Ingredients

- Chicken breasts4–6
- Egg 1
- A cup of almond flour¾ cup
- A grated cup of parmesan cheese¼ cup
- Salt1 ½ tsp
- Black pepper ¼ tsp
- Garlic powder1 tbsp.
- Italian seasoning 2 tsp
- Olive oil 1 tbsp.
- A cup of broccoli florets2 cups
- Salt ½ tsp
- Marinara sauce cup ¼ cup
- Extra parmesan cheese

Instructions

1. The first oven is preheated to 400°. The oven is lined with a baking sheet along with parchment paper. It is then set aside.

2. To a clean shallow bowl, add almond flour, pepper, and parmesan cheese, 1 tsp of salt, garlic powder, and Italian seasoning. Mix all the ingredients well. In a separate dish, add an egg and whisk well.

3. Coat the egg mixture on chicken breasts and then with the almond flour mixture. Set it up in the baking pan.

4. Bake it in the oven for almost 10 minutes. Now remove it from the oven. Just add broccoli. Drizzle some olive oil and the remaining 1/2 tsp of salt over broccoli. Toss it well to coat it. Add on extra parmesan cheese and marinara sauce on top of chicken breast.

5. Again place the pan into the oven for an added 10 minutes until the chicken gets cooked. Cooking time can differ depending on chicken thickness.

Nutrition

Kcal 273, fat 14g, protein 33g,net carbs 14 g

1. Green turmeric tea

Cook time: 5 mins, Servings: 1 cup, Difficulty: easy

Ingredients

- Almond milk(warmed)1¼ cup
- Perfect keto matcha(MCT oil powder)1 scoop
- Cinnamon½ tsp.
- Ground turmeric½–¼ tsp.
- Black pepper (grounded) ¼ tsp.
- Ginger ¼ tsp.
- vanilla flavoring(non-alcoholic) 1 teaspoon
- Stevia/ monk fruit sweetener to taste (optional)

Instructions

1. To a high-speed blender, combine all the ingredients and blend till all the ingredients just mix well.

Nutrition

Kcal 107.5, fat 10.1g, Protein 1g, net carbs 1.5 g

2. Keto protein shake

Cook time: 5 mins, Servings: 1 cup, Difficulty: easy

Ingredients

- Almond milk(unsweetened) 1 cup
- A cup of full-fat coconut milk/ heavy cream 1/4 cup
- Perfect keto chocolate whey protein powder one scoop
- Cacao powder 2 tsp
- Liquid stevia 8–10 drops
- Perfect keto nut butter/ almond butter one teaspoon
- Ice cubes 3–4
- Cacao nibs (optional) 1 tablespoon

- Whipped cream (optional) 2 tablespoons

Instructions

1. Place all the ingredients together and blend until they appear smooth.

2. If preferred, top with Perfect Keto Nut Butter or almond butter, cacao nibs, flakes of coconut, or nuts.

Nutrition

Kcal 273, fat 20g, Protein 17g, net carbs 1.7 g

3. Keto Birthday Cake Shake

Cook time: 5 mins, Servings: 2 cups, Difficulty: easy

Ingredients

- A cup of heavy cream ¼ cup

- A cup of nut milk 1½ cup

- Butter 1tbsp

- Vanilla extract 2 tsp

- Perfect Keto Birthday Cake bar 1

- Swerve/ Lakanto/ keto-friendly sweetener of choice to taste

- Ice (handful)

- Topping(sugar-free sprinkles)

Instructions

1. Add all the required ingredients to a high-speed blender and blend it at high speed until all the ingredients are mixed well.

Nutrition

Kcal 291.3, fat 26.8g, Protein 7.25g, net carbs 3.5 g

4. Chocolate peanut butter smoothie

Cook time: 5 mins, Servings: 2 cups, Difficulty: easy

Ingredients

- almond milk(unsweetened) / low-carb, plant-based milk 1 cup (240 ml)

255

- creamy peanut butter 2tbsp (32g)
- cocoa powder(unsweetened) 1tbsp(4g)
- heavy cream cup 1/4 cup (60 ml)
- a cup of ice 1

Instructions

1. Blend to combine and mix the ingredients in a blender until smooth.

Nutrition

Kcal 345, fat 31g, Protein 11g, net carbs 13 g

5. Coconut blackberry mint smoothie

Cook time: 5 mins, Servings: 1 cup, Difficulty: easy

Ingredients

- Full-fat coconut milk(unsweetened) 1/2 cup
- A cup of frozen blackberries 1/2 cup
- Shredded coconut 2tbsp
- Mint leaves 5-10 leaves

Instructions

1. In a blender, combine and blend until smooth and fluffy.

Nutrition

Kcal 321, fat 29g, Protein 4g, net carbs 17 g

6. Strawberries and cream smoothie

Cook time: 5 mins, Servings: 1 cup, Difficulty: easy

Ingredients

- Water 1/2 cup
- Strawberries froze 1/2 cup
- Heavy cream 1/2 cup

Instructions

1. Take all the ingredients; combine them in a blender until smooth.

Nutrition

Kcal 431, fat 43g, Protein 4g, net carbs 10 g

7. Pumpkin spice smoothie

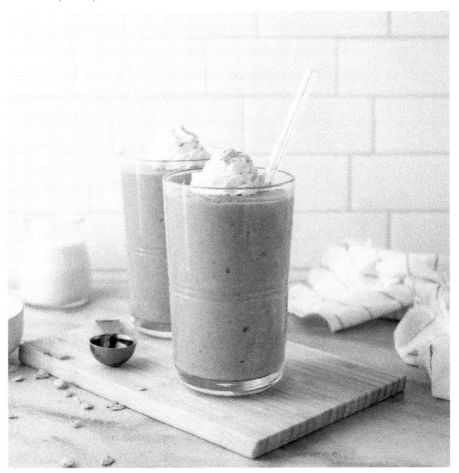

Cook time: 5 mins, Servings: 1 cup, Difficulty: easy

Ingredients

- Unsweetened coconut(unsweetened) / almond milk 1/2 cup

- Pumpkin purée 1/2 cup

- Almond butter 2tbsp

- Pumpkin pie spice ¼ tsp
- A cup of ice 1/2
- Pinch of sea salt

Instructions

1. Take all the ingredients; combine them in a blender until smooth and fluffy.

Nutrition

Kcal 462, fat 42g, Protein 10g, net carbs 19 g

1.   Mashed Cauliflower with Parmesan and Chives

Cook time: 20 mins, Servings: 4-6 cups, Difficulty: easy

Ingredients

- Small heads cauliflower (cored and leaves removed)2 heads
- Chicken broth 2 cups
- Parmesan cheese(grated) 1/4 cup
- Chopped chives (fresh) 1/4 cup
- Kosher salt
- Fresh ground black pepper

Instructions

1.   Add the cauliflower and chicken broth to a medium-sized saucepan, give it a boil. Reduce heat to low. Cover the saucepan and cook for 15 - 20 minutes until the cauliflower becomes tender.

2.   Afterward, with the help of a slotted spoon, shift the cauliflower to a food processor and purée until smooth.

3.   This mixture is then shifted to a bowl and stirred in parmesan and chopped chives. Season it with kosher salt and fresh ground black pepper. Serve it sweet.

Nutrition

Kcal 33, fat 2g, Protein 3g, net carbs 1 g

2.   Curry roasted cauliflower

Cook time: 15 mins, Servings: 4, Difficulty: easy

Ingredients

- Cauliflower(about 2 pounds) 1 head
- Virgin olive oil 1 tbsp. + 1 tsp extra
- Curry powder one ½tsp
- Kosher salt 1tsp

- Lemon juice 2tsp

- Chopped cilantro 1tbsp (to taste)

Instructions

1. First, the oven is preheated to 425° F.

2. Cutaway the outer cauliflower leaves. Split it in half and then cut out and discard the core, which is left out. Slice the cauliflower into parts that are bite-sized. In a deep bowl, cauliflower is tossed with olive oil to coat. Sprinkle with curry powder and salt and cover with a toss. It is then spread out as evenly layered on a large lined and moved into the oven.

3. Roast the cauliflower for about 10 minutes before the bottom starts to tan. Flip it over and continue roasting for more than 5 to 7 minutes till tender. Squeeze the lemon juice and cilantro and toss it all.

Nutrition

Kcal 110, fat 8g, Protein 3g, net carbs 8 g

3. Cauliflower Steaks (roasted) served with Caper M Butter
Cook time: 25 mins, Servings: 4, Difficulty: easy

Ingredients

- Cauliflower (cut into steaks) 1 large head

- Olive oil (as needed) 3-4 tbsp

- Freshly ground black pepper.

- Salt

- Mustard caper browned butter.

- Unsalted butter one stick

- Cloves of garlic(minced) 2

- Coarse-grain mustard 2tbsp

- Drained capers 2tbsp

- Chopped parsley 2tbsp

- Salt

- Ground black pepper(to taste)

Instructions

Cauliflower:

1. To 400 °, the oven is preheated.

2. Over a non-stick baking sheet or aluminum foil, place cauliflower florets or steaks.

3. Brush the cauliflower with olive oil and season properly with salt and black pepper. Let it roast for about 20-25 minutes, turning once.

Brown butter:

1. Butter is placed and melted over medium flame in a saucepan.

2. Reduce the flame and cook for about 5 minutes until caramel color starts appearing, taking care not to burn it.

3. Place it aside now so that the browned bits (milk solids) fall at the end of the pan.

4. Stir in capers, garlic, chopped parsley, mustard. Add to taste, salt, and pepper. Sprinkle over roasted cauliflower and serve warm.

5. It is possible to make butter up to 24 hours in advance. Refrigerate and cool. Reheat gently over low heat in a saucepan.

Nutrition

Kcal 592, fat 8g, Protein 22 g, net carbs 16 g

4. Roasted Vegetables with combination of Moroccan Cauliflower Rice

Cook Time: 50 mins, Servings: 4, Difficulty: capable

Ingredients

- Cauliflower 1

- Mixed peppers(green, yellow, red, and sliced) 3

- Sliced courgettes zucchini 2

- Sliced aubergine 1

- Chopped spring onions 2
- A crushed clove of garlic 1
- Red chili (chopped) 1
- Cumin(grounded) 1 tsp
- Pistachios (roasted) handful
- Parsley(chopped) 50g
- Chopped mint 50g
- A cup of full fat natural yoghurt1/2 cup
- Tahini 2 tbsp.
- Lemon (unwaxed) 1

Instructions

1. First, simply oven is heated to 200 Celsius in advance.

2. Now we slice the peppers, aubergine, and courgettes, leaving back 1/2 red pepper that is thinly sliced and will go into the cauliflower rice.

3. Put in olive oil, toss it, and then add salt and roast for 45-50 minutes. Turn around halfway through.

4. Dry-roast the pistachios now. Simply place them over medium heat in a pan and roast until they are browned. This may take 2 minutes or so. Be careful they aren't burning.

5. Simply blend 150g / 1/2 cup yogurt with two tablespoons of tahini and 1/2 lemon juice in order to make the yogurt tahini sauce. Add a bit of garlic, too, if you like.

6. To make rice for cauliflower, cut off all the outer leaves and the cauliflower into pieces. Cut the rough center out. Next, in the food processor, grate or blitz large chunks until you get rice-sized bits.

7. In a saucepan, just heat one tablespoon of olive oil and add garlic which has been crushed, spring onions nicely chopped, the finely chopped half pepper, and the chopped chili. For 2 minutes, cook it gently.

8. Now add the cauliflower and cook for an additional 5 minutes.

9. Stir in 1 tablespoon of cumin, 1/2 lemon juice, and lemon zest, and also the dry-roasted pistachios.

10. Remove the cauliflower rice from the flame. Now add on the parsley and mint before serving, and combine thoroughly. Add few scattered pomegranate seeds if desired.

11. Organize on one large platter or serve the veggies and rice separately on two plates.

12. The dish tastes pretty good, hot or cold.

Nutrition

Kcal 147, fat 7.4g, Protein 6.8g, net carbs 17.8 g

5. Cauliflower rice with garlic and green onion

Cook time: 30 mins, Servings: 4, Difficulty: easy

Ingredients

- Cauliflower pieces(stems included) 4 heaping cups
- Olive oil2 t
- Cloves of garlic(cut in half) big eight cloves
- Sliced green onion 1 cup
- Salt(to taste)
- Black pepper (fresh and grounded to taste)
- For using a 12 oz. Bag of riced cauliflower
- Riced cauliflower 12 oz.
- Olive oil 1 1/2 t
- Cloves of garlic 5-6
- Green onion(sliced) 3/4 cup
- Salt (to taste)
- Fresh black pepper (to taste)

Instructions

1. Slice the cauliflower into smaller pieces of the same size until four generous cups of pieces of cauliflower, including the stems, are ready.

2. Process 2 cups of cauliflower pieces at the moment in the food processor using the steel blade, buzzing it in short bursts until it is finely chopped enough, but slightly larger, to resemble rice.

3. Open the bag of cauliflower if available.

4. The garlic cloves are peeled and then slice them lengthwise in half.

5. Chop sufficient green onions for the amount of cauliflower we have.

6. Oil is heated over a low flame in a non-stick frying pan until it feels hot, then put the garlic cloves and stir-fry until garlic smell could be sensed.

7. The moment there is the slightest color change in the garlic, remove the garlic and discard.

8. Now put the cauliflower in the hot pan while season it with salt and freshly ground black pepper.

9. Fry the cauliflower and turn it over regularly until it starts to soften and lose the raw flavor, around 3-4 minutes.

10. Turn off the flame, add the green onions, and serve right away.

Nutrition

Kcal 181, fat 13g, Protein 5g, net carbs 7.6 g

6. Cauliflower Cheese & Onion Croquette

Cook time: 15 mins, servings: 12 croquettes, Difficulty: medium

Ingredients

- Cauliflower 1
- parmesan cheese (grated) 1 cup
- Garlic powder 2tsp
- Spring onions(chopped) 4
- Cheddar cheese grated 1/2 cup

- Dijon mustard1/2 tsp
- Salt ½ tsp
- Pepper ½ tsp
- Olive oil 2tbsp

Instructions

1. First, the cauliflower is chopped into florets, put in a water pan, bring it to a boil, cover, and simmer until soft for 10-15 minutes.
2. Now drain the water and let it cool.
3. Draw out the excess water from the florets by squeezing.
4. Mash the cauliflower by using a hand or with a blender.
5. Add the remaining spring onions, 1 cup of Parmesan cheese, Cheddar cheese, mustard, and seasoning. Thoroughly blend.
6. Make croquettes shapes by using your hand.
7. Layer the croquettes on parchment/greaseproof paper and place them in the refrigerator for about 30 minutes.
8. Now on a frying pan, heat the olive oil over a medium flame.
9. Fry the croquettes softly, turning over until the color is golden.
10. Ready to eat and enjoy.

Nutrition

Kcal 86, fat 6g, Protein 5g, net carbs 2.6 g

7. Roasted Garlic-Parmesan Zucchini, Squash, and Tomatoes

Cook time: 30 mins, Servings: 6 servings, Difficulty: medium

Ingredients

- Small zucchini (half an inch thick slices) 2
- Yellow squash (small sized) (half an inch slice) 2
- Flavoring /small tomatoes (Campari) 14 oz
- Olive oil 3tbp
- Minced cloves of garlic 4

- Italian seasoning one and a half tsp
- Salt and black pepper(grounded)
- Shredded parmesan cheese a full cup(2.4 oz)
- Fresh/ parsley dried (for garnish)

Instructions

1. First, we preheat the oven to a temperature of 400 °. Line the oven with an 18 by 13-inch rimmed baking sheet along with aluminum foil or a sheet of parchment paper. Altogether whisk the garlic, olive oil, and also the remaining Italian seasoning in a bowl (let it rest for a time of 5 - 10 minutes if possible so that flavors absorb into oil). In another bowl, put the zucchini, tomatoes and squash altogether. Pour the mixture of olive oil over the top and toss gently with your hands to blend evenly.

2. Pour onto a fully prepared baking dish and distribute it evenly. With the combination of salt and some amount of pepper, season it. Sprinkle each top with parmesan. Roast 25 - 30 minutes in a preheated oven till the veggies are soft and tender, and the parmesan gets golden brown in color. If desired, garnish it with some parsley and serve hot.

Nutrition

Kcal 168, fat 11g, Protein 5g, net carbs 8 g

8. Bacon & smoked gouda cauliflower mash (low carb and gluten free)

Cook time: 20 mins, Servings: 3 cups, Difficulty: easy

Ingredients

- Cauliflower florets 4 cups
- Heavy cream 3tbsp
- Butter 2tbsp
- Kosher salt 1/2 tsp
- Black pepper 1/4 tsp
- Garlic powder 1/4 tsp

- Cooked bacon four slices
- Smoked gouda cheese(shredded) 1/3 cup
- Salt (to taste)
- Pepper(to taste)

Instructions

1. In the microwave dish, the cauliflower, garlic powder, heavy cream, butter, salt, and pepper are placed. Microwave them all for 18 to 20 minutes until soft. Move the liquid and cauliflower to a food processor. Further, add the bacon and the smoked Gouda in it. Blend until creamy and smooth. As needed, season with additional pinch of salt and some pepper

Nutrition

Kcal 282, fat 22g, Protein 12g, net carbs 6 g

Chapter 7: Vegan recipes

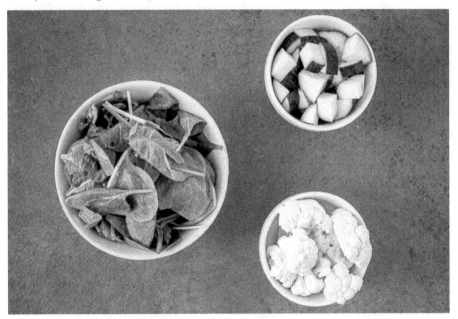

1. Smoothie Bowl (low carb) with Cauliflower and Greens

Cook time: 15 mins, Servings: 2, Difficulty: easy

Ingredients

- Frozen cauliflower1/2 cup

- Frozen zucchini1/2 cup

- Frozen spinach 1 cup

- Frozen blueberries 1 cup

- A cup of milk 1 cup

- Almond butter/peanut butter2 tbsp

- Hemp hearts3 tbsp

- Cinnamon (grounded)1 tsp

- Optional toppings

- Berries (fresh /frozen)

- Granola (grain-free)

Instructions

1. This bowl of smoothie fits best with frozen cauliflower and zucchini. The choice of steaming the cauliflower first, but this move is not required when using a high-speed blender such as a Vitamix. It's convenient to have frozen spinach, but fresh works fine as well.

2. We combine all of the ingredients in a blender, beginning with the frozen ingredients close to the blade. Blend till a creamy consistency is obtained and all the ingredients are well integrated.

3. The banana-free smoothie bowl mix should be split into two bowls. Homemade granola, new fruit, and extra hemp hearts are used for topping.

4. Try to steam a big batch of it in the freezer and store it.

Nutrition

Kcal 253, fat 14.8g, Protein 12g, net carbs 18.5 g

2. Best ever guacamole

Cook time: 10 mins, Servings: 4, Difficulty: easy

Ingredients

- Avocados(ripe) 3
- Onion(small and finely diced) 1/2
- Roma tomatoes(nicely diced) 2
- Fresh cilantro(chopped) 3tbsp
- Jalapeno pepper(seeds removed) 1
- Garlic cloves(minced) 2 cloves
- Lime(juiced) 1
- Sea salt ½ tsp

Instructions

1. In a large bowl, chop the avocados in half, remove out the pit and scoop out.
2. Avocado is scooped into a mixing bowl.
3. With the help of a fork, avocado is mashed, and it is made as chunky or smooth as you would like.
4. Mix and stir together the remaining ingredients. Try giving it a taste test and, if necessary, add a little bit more salt or lime juice.
5. Now plate the guacamole with tortilla chips.
6. Guacamole next to tortilla chips is served.

Nutrition

Kcal 184.8, fat 15.8g, Protein 2.5g, net carbs 12.3 g

3. Maple low carb oatmeal

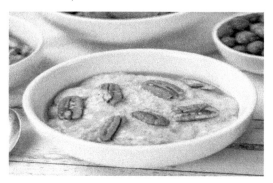

Cook Time: 20 mins, Servings: 4, Difficulty: easy

Ingredients

- Walnuts(1/2 cups)
- Pecans(1/2 cups)
- Sunflower seeds (1/4 cups)
- Coconut flakes (1/4 cups)
- Almond milk(unsweetened) 4 cups
- Chia seeds 4tbsp
- Stevia powder3/8 tsp
- Cinnamon1/2 tsp
- maple flavoring (optional)1 tsp

Instructions

1. In a food processor, add the walnuts, sunflower seeds, and pecans and pulse them a few times to crumble.

2. Add all of the ingredients into a big pot. Stir on low and simmer for a reasonable 20-30 minutes, until most of the liquid has been absorbed by the chia seeds. Don't forget to stir, as the seeds will stick to the bottom of the jar.

3. Turn down the heat when the oatmeal appears thickened and serve warm. It can also be cooled down and stored the next day in the refrigerator for breakfast.

4. End up serving with fresh fruit and any other toppings needed.

Nutrition

Kcal 374, fat 34.59g, Protein 9.25g, net carbs 3.274 g

4. Vegan Arugula Avocado Tomato Salad

Cook time: 20 mins, Servings: 8, Difficulty: easy

Ingredients

- Arugula Salad
- Baby arugula(chopped roughly) 5 oz
- Large basil leaves (sliced) 6 leaves
- Pint yellow grape tomatoes half sliced.
- Pint red grape tomatoes half sliced.
- Large avocados(chunks) 2
- Red onion (minced) 1/2 cup
- Balsamic Vinaigrette
- Balsamic vinegar 2 tbsp
- Olive oil 1tbsp
- Maple syrup 1 tbsp
- Juice of lemon 1 tbsp
- Garlic clove(minced) 1
- Himalayan pink sea salt 1/4 tsp
- Black pepper 1/4 tsp

Instructions

1. Put the roughly chopped arugula and sliced basil leaves into a large mixing bowl. Add the sliced grape tomatoes, avocado chunks, and minced red onion to the bowl. Toss to combine.

2. Put into a large mixing bowl the finely chopped arugula and basil leaves which have been sliced. Add to the bowl the sliced grape tomatoes, chunks of avocado, and minced red onion. Now toss it to combine.

3. Now the balsamic dressing is poured over the salad. Mix the salad carefully until the dressing is uniformly distributed, and then moves the salad to a large bowl.

Note

- Chop the arugula roughly so it is bite-sized.

- Wait until you serve to add the avocado if you are making this vegan arugula salad to bring to a dinner. If the avocado chunks are added too early, they may begin to turn brown. Add few drops of lemon juice over the avocado chunks if you have to add the avocado early to prevent them from turning brown.

- For this salad, use avocados that are firm with only a little bit of giving when pressing them. If the avocado is sufficiently soft for guacamole, then this is too ripe for the dish. Avocado should retain its shape when tossed.

- If the avocados are a little soft, dice them instead of mixing them into the salad and top the salad with them. This way, once you toss it, the avocado will not break down and become too mushy in the salad.

- Store it for 1-2 days in an airtight jar in the fridge if there is some leftover arugula salad. The next day, that salad won't be as fresh, but it would still be edible. When about to eat it, add a little bit of fresh arugula to the leftovers to freshen it up.

Nutrition

Kcal 134, fat 9g, Protein 3g, net carbs 12 g

5. Vegan Sesame Ginger Coleslaw

Cook time: 15 mins, Servings: 12 servings, Difficulty: easy

Ingredients

- Sesame Ginger Dressing -
- Almond butter2 tbsp.
- Tahini 1tbsp.
- Low-sodium tamari2 tbsp.
- Rice vinegar2 tbsp.
- Lime (juice) 3tbsp.
- Hot sauce 1tbsp.
- Maple syrup 1tbsp.
- Medium clove of garlic (peeled) 1
- Fresh ginger (peeled) 2-inch knob

Coleslaw -

- Green cabbage(sliced thinly) 5 cups
- Red cabbage(sliced thinly) 5 cups
- Carrots (sliced thinly) 2 cups
- Cilantro (roughly chopped) 1 cup
- Green onions (sliced) 1 cup

Instructions

1. Put two tablespoons of almond butter, one tablespoon of tahini, two tablespoons of rice vinegar, two tablespoons of tamari, three tablespoons of lime juice, one tablespoon of hot sauce, one tablespoon of maple syrup, one clove of garlic, and a 2" knob of ginger into just a small mixing cup. Blend until smooth, thick, and creamy.

2. Place into a bowl and mix the red and green cabbage thinly sliced, cilantro, carrots, and green onions. Now pour dressing over the mixture of cabbage and toss it to blend.

3. Put the coleslaw in the fridge and cover it before placing inside. Chill for 1 hour.

Note

- For saving time and make this vegan coleslaw even simpler, use a pack of pre-shredded carrots.

- Salt the cabbage so that slaw doesn't get soggy before dressing it to draw out the excess liquid in case of few days in the fridge. It is an additional move, but it is worth the effort.

- Using a spoon to peel the skin off of the ginger knob, cut off the slice of ginger that is to be used for the dressing. In an airtight jar, place the peeled ginger and store that in the freezer. For months, it will remain fresh, and freezing the ginger makes it really easy to grate.

- Keep the leftover coleslaw for 3-5 days in the fridge in an airtight jar.

Nutrition

Kcal 66, fat 2g, Protein 3g, net carbs 11 g

6. Lemon Garlic Oven Roasted Asparagus

Cook time: 12 mins, Servings: 4 servings, Difficulty: easy

Ingredients

- Asparagus (about 25-30 stalks) 1 lb
- Olive oil1 tbsp.
- Dried thyme1/4 tsp
- Onion granules 1/4 tsp
- Lemon zest1 tsp
- Himalayan sea salt and pepper(to taste)
- Lemon slices 4-5
- Cloves of garlic(minced)
- Olive oil 1 tsp
- Fresh lemon juice 1 tbsp.

- Vegan parmesan cheese 1-2 tbsp.

Instructions

1. The oven is preheated to 425 ° first.

2. Wash and dry the asparagus quite well. Prep the asparagus: Wash and dry the asparagus quite well. Either bend the asparagus in half part and let it snap normally, or cut off the base of the stalk by 1 to 1 1/2 inches.

3. Spread the asparagus spears on a tray lined with parchment. Drizzle the asparagus with over 1 tbsp. Olive oil and stir to coat each slice. Sprinkle uniformly over the asparagus following ingredients: thyme, onion granules, pepper, sea salt, and lemon zest, and toss it for one more time. Use lemon slices to top and bake for 8 minutes.

4. Mince the cloves of garlic and place them into the bowl. Take one teaspoon of olive oil and blend it together. Take off the tray from the oven after cooking the asparagus for 8 minutes and spread the minced garlic uniformly over the tray. Take the tray back in the oven and bake for an additional 3-4 minutes.

5. When the asparagus gets tender and not mushy, remove it from the tray. The color should still be bright green.   Over the asparagus, squeeze the half lemon juice (about 1 tbsp.) and top it with finely grated vegan parmesan cheese.

Note

- For this recipe, use one whole lemon. Next, zest the lemon using a Micro plane. Then slice the lemon in half and set aside one half for the juice, and then cut the other half for garnish.

- 1 /2 tsp of garlic powder can be substituted for the additional step of adding the fresh minced garlic.

- Do not add the fresh garlic too soon, and it will burn and taste very bitter if you're doing it.

- Cut off the woody sides of the asparagus before roasting.

- If lemon juice is added before cooking, instead of roasting, the asparagus can steam into the liquid. It's always going to taste fine, but not going to get those tasty little crispy edges.

- Be cautious not to overcook the asparagus; continue to check it. If it's not bright green upon picking it up, it's soft and bendy; then it's probably overcooked.

Nutrition

Kcal 67, fat 4g, Protein 2g, net carbs 5 g

6. Paleo broccoli fried rice (whole30, keto)

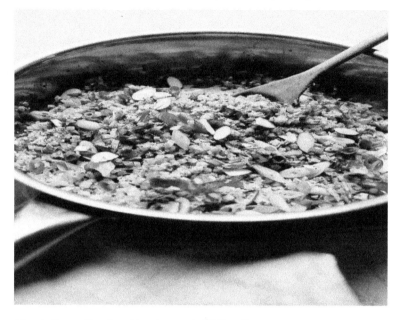

Cook time: 3 mins, Servings: 4, Difficulty: easy

Ingredients

- Two heads riced broccoli 4 cups.
- Ghee/ avocado oil1 tbsp.
- Finely Chopped garlic1 tbsp.
- Coconut aminos1 tbsp.
- Toasted sesame oil1.5 tsp
- Coarse salt(to taste)
- Frozen ginger(grated) ¼ - ½ tsp
- A quarter of one lime juice (more for serving)
- Scallions(chopped)2 bulbs
- Chopped cilantro/ parsley (optional) 4tbsp.
- Sprinkle with sliced almonds (optional)
- Optional pairings:

- Scallops (fresh) 8-10
- Medium-sized shrimp(peeled and uncooked) ½ lb
- Coarse salt¼ tsp
- Black pepper⅛ tsp

Instructions

1. Add one tablespoon of ghee to a well-heated skillet. Sauté the riced broccoli in a pan for 1 min along with finely chopped garlic. In order to season riced broccoli, add coconut amino, toasted sesame oil, and coarse salt. Sauté for an extra 2 mins. Broccoli should be cooked until the color is bright green.

2. Take it off the heat and grate about half a teaspoon of frozen ginger over the rice while the broccoli rice will still be warm. It is then seasoned with some lime juice.

3. Now garnish this with scallions, sliced almonds, and cilantro. Serve on the side with additional lime wedges.

Nutrition

Kcal 87, fat 5g, Protein 2g, net carbs 7 g

7. Roasted Vegetable Tofu Tacos

Cook time: 70 minutes, Servings: 10 tofu servings, Difficulty: capable

Ingredients

Roasted Vegetables

- Medium cauliflower 1
- Sliced cremini mushrooms ½ lb
- Bell peppers medium (sliced) 2
- Chili powder 1 tsp
- Cumin 1 tsp
- Onion powder 1 tsp
- Powder of garlic 1 tsp
- Smoked paprika 1 tsp
- Salt ¼ tsp

- Black pepper ¼ tsp

Crumbled Tofu

- Vegetable broth/ water ¼ cup (to sauté)
- Firm tofu (pressed) 1 package
- Red onion medium (diced) 1
- Cloves of garlic (minced) 3
- Tomato paste 1 tbsp.
- Worcestershire sauce 1 tbsp.
- Chili powder 1 tbsp.
- Paprika 1 tbsp.
- Cumin 1 tbsp.
- Salt ¼ tsp
- Black pepper ¼ tsp

Taco Ingredients

- Spinach tortillas 8
- Head butter lettuce 1
- Avocado (sliced/large) 1
- Hot sauce

Instructions

1. To extract excess liquid, squeeze the tofu into a press for about 30 minutes. One can also cover the tofu block in a dish towel if there is no available press and put a heavy container on top of it.
2. Roasted Vegetables
3. Firstly get the oven preheated to 400 degrees.
4. Upon two big silicone-lined trays, organize the cauliflower florets, sliced mushrooms, and then sliced bell peppers.
5. Sprinkle the vegetables with chili powder, garlic powder, onion powder, smoked paprika, cumin, salt, and black pepper and

toss generously to coat. Now bake it for duration of 30 minutes or till all is soft and the tips of the cauliflower florets are of light brown color.

Crumbled Tofu

1. Place the pan over medium heat; while the vegetables get roasted, sauté the chopped red onion in the vegetable broth until it gets soft and translucent in appearance. If the pan looks too dry, add more liquid.

2. The minced garlic, tomato paste, and vegan Worcestershire sauce should be added next. Place it on the heat for an additional 2 minutes while stirring.

3. Move everything else to one side of tray and crumble the block of pressed tofu around the other side of the saucepan with your hands. Sprinkle over the tofu with chili powder, smoked paprika, pepper, cumin, and salt. Stir the tofu to coat with seasonings and then mix together all in the pan. Reduce the heat down to medium-low and cook the mixture for at least about 10 minutes, frequently stirring until thoroughly warmed.

4. The roasted vegetables must be prepared at the same time as the mixture of tofu is ready. Low-carb wraps, roasted vegetables, lettuce, butter, a scoop of tofu crumbles, avocado slices, and a splash of hot sauce make the tacos.

Note

- Try using a firm or extra-firm tofu for the best texture.

- To have a dry or form texture, press and drain the tofu before transferring to the pan and thus have a dry, firm texture.

- Try to stop overcrowding the sheet pans. The vegetables will only steam instead of roasting if the pan is too crowded.

- Keep the leftover filling for 4-5 days in an airtight jar in the fridge or freeze it for a later meal.

Nutrition

Kcal 118, fat 5g, Protein 7g, net carbs 13 g

8. Keto Roasted Radishes

Cook time: 30 minutes, Servings: 6 servings, Difficulty: easy

Ingredients

- Radishes 20-25
- Vegetable broth 1/2 cup
- Medium cloves of garlic(minced) 3
- Dried rosemary1/2 tsp
- onion powder1/2 tsp
- Dried oregano1/4 tsp
- Salt1/4 tsp
- Black pepper1/4 tsp
- Fresh rosemary one sprig (optional)

Instructions

1. Firstly the oven is preheated to 400°.
2. By cutting off the leaves, greens, and roots, prepare the radishes. Well, rinse them. Then slice every radish in half. Quarter them so that they cook quickly if the radishes are any larger than a quarter.
3. Now pour the vegetable broth and add minced garlic, rosemary, oregano, salt, black pepper, and onion powder into a standard size baking dish. To mix the seasonings, whisk it well.
4. Transfer all the radishes to a baking dish, spoon the broth over each one of the radishes to coat, and afterward cover and bake for about 30-35 minutes (check whether the radishes are on the small side for 25 minutes) or until the radishes are soft, stirring midway through.
5. Garnish prior to serving with new rosemary. Place the leftovers for about 4-5 days in an airtight jar in the refrigerator.

Note

- Should choose those radishes that seem to be similar in size so that they are evenly roasted.

- Should roast the raw vegetables in a casserole dish so they remain hydrated since they are not coated in oil while roasting.

- Place the leftovers for 4-5 days in an airtight jar in the fridge.

Nutrition

Kcal 25, fat 1g, Protein 1g, net carbs 1 g

9. Vegan Garlic Aioli

Cook time: 5 mins, Servings: 8 servings, Difficulty: easy

Ingredients

- A cup of original veganaise 3/4 cup

- Garlic cloves medium (minced) 3

- Lemon juice about 2.5 tbsp.

- Himalayan pink sea salt 1/4 tsp

- Black pepper 1/4 tsp

Instructions

1. In a bowl, add all the ingredients and use a whisk to mix. Now cover and refrigerate prior to serving for 30 minutes.

2. Note

3. Press the palm strongly on top of the lemon before cutting the lemon and roll it back and forth to loosen up the juice.

4. If possible, use fresh garlic to add more flavor than dried seasonings.

5. Place the leftover aioli for 5-7 days in an airtight jar in the fridge.

6. Need not freeze the remaining vegan garlic aioli because it does not have the same consistency as the vegan mayo separates.

Nutrition

Kcal 138, fat 14g, Protein 1g, net carbs 2 g

1. Paleo (low carb) cinnamon sugar donuts

Cook time: 15 mins, Servings: 12mini donuts, Difficulty: easy

Ingredients

- Eggs (room temp) 2 large
- Almond milk (unsweetened) 1/4 cup
- Apple cider vinegar 1/4 tsp
- Vanilla extract 1tsp
- Melted ghee 2tbsp
- Granulated monk fruit sweetener /swerve 1/4 cup.
- Blanched almond flour(fine) 1 cup
- Coconut flour ½ tbsp.
- Xanthan gum ¼ tsp
- Ground cinnamon 1tsp
- Baking powder one half tsp
- Sodium bicarbonate(Baking soda) half tsp
- Sea salt 1/8

Topping choices:

For the Cinnamon Sugar Coating:

- Granulated monk fruit /granulated erythritol /swerve 1/4 cup
- Ground cinnamon 1tsp
- Melted ghee / butter 1 1/2 tablespoons
- For the Chocolate Glaze:
- Dark chocolate (sugarless) melted 2 ounces.
- Coconut oil 1tsp
- Powdered monk fruit sweetener 1tsp

Instructions

1. Whisk the eggs, almond milk, vanilla, apple cider vinegar, melted ghee, melted ghee & monk fruit sweetener altogether in a large mixing bowl, until smooth and mixed.

2. Combine the almond and coconut flour, baking powder, xanthan gum, cinnamon, some sodium bicarbonate, and salt in an individual medium dish. Now mix the remaining ingredients to the wet components slowly and mix until they are just blended.

3. Uniformly shift batter into a greased mini donut pan of 12 cavity silicone.

4. Now bake to a preheated 350F oven for 12-15 minutes till we have the golden brown color there.

5. Put off the pan from oven & carefully remove it until it is cool enough to touch the donuts.

For the cinnamon coating:

1. Stir the granulated sweetener and cinnamon together in a shallow dish while the donuts are baking.

2. Melt ghee in a smaller sized heat-safe cup.

3. Now take over each cooling donut and dip lightly in melted ghee, after which roll into the cinnamon/sweetener's coating.

4. Redo this with the rest of the donuts.

For the chocolate glaze:

1. To a small heat-safe mug, add the finely chopped chocolate and coconut oil & melt them in the microwave. Add the sweetener until mixed.

2. Now the cooled donuts are dipped into the chocolate and put in the refrigerator till the chocolate coating is set.

Nutrition

Kcal 86, fat 8g, Protein 2g, net carbs 2 g

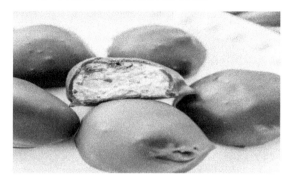

Cook time: 20 mins, Serving: 18, Difficulty: easy

Ingredients

- Salted peanuts chopped 1 cup.

- Peanut butter 1 cup

- Powdered sweetener such as swerve

- Sugar-free chocolate chips 8 oz.

Instructions

1. Mix the sliced peanuts, peanut butter, and the sweetener altogether. Distribute the 18-piece dough and shape it into balls. Place them on a baking sheet lined with wax paper. Refrigerate it until cold.

2. In the microwave or on top of the double boiler, melt the chips of chocolate chips. Let the chocolate chips stay in the microwave, stirring every other 30 seconds unless they are 75% melted. And then just stir until the rest of it melts.

3. Now each ball of peanut butter is dipped into the chocolate, and bring it back on the wax paper. Until the chocolate sets, put it in the fridge.

Nutrition

Kcal 194, fat 17g, Protein 7g, net carbs 7 g

3. Keto Sopapilla Cheesecake Bars

Cook time: 50mins, Servings: 16 bars, Difficulty: capable

Ingredients

Dough Ingredients:

- Mozzarella shredded/ cubed 8 oz.
- Cream cheese 2 oz.
- Egg 1
- Almond flour 1/3 cup
- Coconut flour 1/3 cup
- Joy filled eats sweetener 2 tbsp.
- Vanilla 1 tsp
- Baking powder 1 tsp

Cheesecake Filling Ingredients:

- Cream cheese 14 oz.
- Eggs 2
- Joy filled eats sweetener ½ cups.
- Vanilla 1 tsp
- Cinnamon Topping:
- Joy-Filled Eats Sweetener 2 tbsp.
- Cinnamon 1 tbsp.
- Butter (melted) 2 tbsp.

Instructions

1. First, we pre-set the oven and heat it to 350.
2. Place cheese in a bowl that is microwave-safe. Place for one minute in a microwave. Yeah, stir. Microwave it for 30-second. Stir again. All the cheese ought to be melted at this stage. Microwave it for about 30 more seconds before uniform and gloopy (it should be like cheese fondue in appearance at this point). Add in the food processor, the remainder of the dough ingredients and the cheese. Mix until a uniform hue by using a dough blade. Wet your hands when it is uniform in color and put

half of it into an 8x8 baking dish. On the piece of parchment paper, press the other remaining half into an 8x8 rectangle.

3.   Now add the cream cheese, vanilla, eggs, and then sweetener to the food processor to start making the cheesecake filling. Mix into the food processor/ electric blender until smooth.

4.   Now the cheesecake batter is poured on top of the bottom part of the dough. Place over the other piece of dough gently on top and peel the parchment paper off. Sprinkle the cinnamon and sweetener on the top of it and glaze with the melted butter.

5.   Bake till it is puffed up and golden brown in color, for about 50-60 minutes. Brush over the top with the help of a pastry brush over the last 20 minutes of baking if the butter collects in the middle.

Nutrition

Kcal 190, fat 16g, Protein 6g, net carbs 4 g

4.   Best Keto Brownies

Cook Time: 20 mins, Servings: 16 brownies, Difficulty: easy

Ingredients

- 1/2 cup
- Three quarter cup
- 3/4 cup
- 1/2 tsp baking powder
- One tablespoon instant coffee optional
- 10 tablespoons butter (or 1/2 cup + 2 Tblsp)
- 2 oz dark chocolate
- Three eggs at room temperature
- ½ teaspoon optional

Instructions

1.   Set the oven, preheated to 350 degrees. Now place an 8x8 inch or 8x9 pan with the layer of aluminum foil, parchment paper, or grease it with butter.

2. Whisk and blend the almond flour, cocoa powder, baking powder together along with erythritol and instant coffee in a mixing cup of medium size. Better make sure that whisk out almost all the clumps of erythritol.

3. Melt the butter and chocolate in a broad microwave-safe bowl and let it stay for about 30 seconds - 1 minute or till it melts. Whisk in the vanilla and eggs and then gradually stir in the dry ingredients until mixed. Be careful not to mix the batter over for a long time, or it's going to get cakey.

4. Move the batter to a baking dish and bake for about 18-20 minutes or until the inserted toothpick comes out wet. Cool in the refrigerator for at least about 30 minutes to 2 hours, and then slice into 16 smaller pieces.

Nutrition

Kcal 116, fat 11g, Protein 2g, net carbs 3 g

5. White Chocolate Peanut Butter Blondies

Cook time: 25 mins, Servings: 16 blondies, Difficulty: easy

Ingredients

- Peanut butter ½ cup

- Butter (Softened) 4 tbsp.

- Eggs 2

- Vanilla 1 tsp

- Raw cocoa butter (Melted) 3 tbsp.

- Almond flour ¼ cup

- Coconut flour 1 tbsp.

- Joy filled eats sweetener ½ cups.

- Cup of raw cocoa (chopped) ¼ cup

Instructions

1. At first, the oven is heated to 350. Then cooking spray is sprayed on the base of a 9 x 9 baking dish.

2. Blend the very first five ingredients via an electric mixer until smooth. Flour, sweetener, and chopped cocoa butter are added. Arrange on a baking dish. Bake for about 25 minutes till the middle no more jiggles, and the edges are golden brown in color.

3. Cool properly, and then chill for at least 2-3 hours in the refrigerator before cutting.

4. Note

5. Use the blend of xylitol, erythritol, and stevia, which is twice as sweet as sugar.

6. Very concentrated sweeteners in this recipe do not work.

Nutrition

Kcal 103, fat 9g, Protein 3g, net carbs 2 g

6. Keto Blueberry Lemon Cheesecake Bars

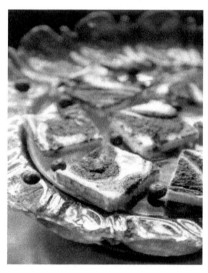

Cook time: 20 mins, Servings: 12, Difficulty: easy

Ingredients

Almond Flour Crust

- butter 8tbsp
- almond flour 1 1/4 cup

- swerve sweetener 2tbsp
- Low Carb Blueberry Sauce
- blueberries 1 1/2 cup
- water 1/4 cup
- confectioners swerve sweetener 1/3 cup
- Lemon Cheesecake Layer
- block cream cheese 1/8 ounce
- egg yolk 1
- confectioners swerve 1/3 cup
- lemon juice 1tbsp
- lemon zest(packed) 1tsp
- vanilla extract 1tsp

Coconut Crumble Topping

- Butter 2tbsp
- Almond flour 1/4 cup
- Coconut flakes(unsweetened) 1/4 cup
- Swerve sweetener 1tbsp

Instructions

1. To start preparing the Blueberry Sauce, add blueberries, sweetener, and water to swerve. Enable the mixture to boil for approximately 10-15 minutes before it becomes thick. Place aside.

2. An oven is preheated for the crust at 350 degrees.

3. Through a foil or parchment paper, cover an 8x8 sheet.

4. Combine in a mixing bowl the melted butter, almond flour and swerve and drop into the pan lined with foil.

5. Prebake crust for about 7 minutes. It must not be firm, only starting to get brown around the edges slightly.

6. Remove and allow the crust to cool. While it is hot, DO NOT add the cheesecake layer.

For the Lemon Cheesecake Layer:

1. Blend in the cream cheese, the yolk of egg, sweetener, and lemon juice, zest, and remove until fluffy and smooth by using an electric mixer.

2. Spread the layer of cheesecake uniformly over the crust.

For the Blueberry Layer:

1. Over through the cheesecake mixture, pour the made low carb blueberry sauce.

For the Crumble:

1. In a blender/ food processor, mix butter, almond flour, unsweetened coconut, and sweetener and also process till it represents a mixture-like crumb.

2. Spread over the blueberry layer over it.

3. Bake until the top is lightly brown in color for 18-20 minutes.

4. Enable the bars to cool before slicing fully.

Note

- To get nice clean slices, put the bars in the freezer for 15 minutes prior to slicing.

Nutrition Facts

Kcal 256, fat 19.9g, Protein 4g, net carbs 6.6 g

7. Espresso chocolate cheesecake bars

Cook time: 35 mins, Servings: 16, Difficulty: medium

Ingredients

For the chocolate crust:

- Butter(melted) 7tbsp

- Blanched almond flour 2 cups

- Cocoa powder 3tbsp

- Granulated erythritol sweetener 1/3 cup

- For the cheesecake:
- Full fat cream cheese 16 ounces
- Big eggs 2
- Granulated erythritol sweetener 1/2 cup
- Espresso instant powder 2 tbsp
- Vanilla extract 1 tsp
- Cocoa powder for dusting.

Instructions

The chocolate crust:

1. Preheat the oven to 350° F.
2. Combine the cocoa powder, melted butter, almond flour, and sweetener in a medium-sized dish and blend nicely.
3. Shift the crust of dough to a 9 x 9 pan.
4. Place the crust to the bottom of the dish.
5. The crust is then baked for 8 minutes.
6. Take it off from the oven and set it aside to cool.

Cheesecake filling:

1. Combine the espresso powder, cream cheese, sweetener, eggs, and vanilla extract in a blender and blend until smooth.
2. The crust is poured over the par-baked crust and spread out uniformly into the pan.
3. Bake the cheesecake bars at 350° F for 25 minutes, or until set.
4. Remove from the oven and cool.
5. Dust with optional cocoa powder if using.
6. Chill for at least 1 hour, and cut into four rows of squares to serve.
7. Store in an air-tight container in the refrigerator for up to 5 days, or freeze for up to 3 months.

Nutrition

Kcal 232, fat 21g, Protein 6g, net carbs 5 g

8.   Pressure Cooker Keto Ricotta Lemon Cheesecake

Cook time: 40 mins, Servings: 6, Difficulty: medium

Ingredients

- Cream Cheese 8 oz.
- Truvia 1/4 cup
- Ricotta cheese 1/3 cup
- Zest of lemon 1
- Lemon Juice 1/4 cup
- Lemon Extract 1/2
- Eggs 2

For topping

- Sour cream 2tbsp
- Truvia 1tsp

Instructions

1. Use a stand mixer; blend all ingredients, excluding the eggs, till a smooth mixture with no granules is left.
2. Now taste it to verify the sweet according to liking.
3. Put the two eggs, deduce the speed and blend gently until the eggs are added. Over-beating can result in a cracked crust at this point.
4. Place into a 6-inch spring-form oiled pan and wrap in foil or a silicone lid.
5. Put two water cups and a trivet in the inner liner of the Instant Pot. Position the foil-covered bowl on the trivet.
6. Cook about 30 minutes at high pressure, and allow it to release the pressure gradually.
7. Combine and spread the sour cream and Truvia on the warm cake.
8. Now refrigerate it for about 6-8 hours.

Oven Instructions

- Prepare the ingredients for the cheesecake as described in the Instant Pot directions.
- Create a water bath and put the pan with the ingredients for the cheesecake inside.
- Bake for about 35 minutes at 375F.

Nutrition

Kcal 181, fat 16g, Protein 5g, net carbs 2 g

9. Keto Ginger Cookie Recipe

Cook time: 15 mins, Servings: 18 cookies, Difficulty: easy

Ingredients

- Cream Together
- Butter/ coconut oil (softened) 4 tbsp.
- Agave nectar 2 tbsp.
- Eggs 1
- Water 2tbsp
- Add Dry Ingredients
- Superfine Almond Flour 2.5 cup
- Truvia/sugar 1/3 cup
- Ground ginger 2tsp
- Ground Cinnamon 1 tsp
- Ground Nutmeg 0.5 tsp
- Baking Soda 1 tsp
- Kosher Salt 0.25 tsp

Instructions

1. First, get the oven preheated to 350F.
2. Now line the baking pan with parchment paper and set it aside.
3. Mix butter, agave nectar, egg, and water altogether.

4. Transfer all the dried ingredients to this mixture and blend well at a reduced speed.

5. Now roll into 2 tsp balls and place them on a baking tray which is lined with parchment paper. They just don't spread too far, but they leave a little gap between them.

6. Bake till the tops become lightly brown in color for about 12-15 minutes.

7. Keep in an air-tight jar when cooled. For, like, an hour before you eat them all, cookies would be around.

Nutrition

Kcal 122, fat 10g, Protein 3g, net carbs 5 g

10. Cream Cheese Pound Cake | Keto Pound Cake

Cook time: 40, Servings: 8, Difficulty: easy

Ingredients

- Cream Cheese(room temperature) 4 ounces
- Softened butter 4tbsp
- Swerve / Truvia 0.5 cup
- Almond Extract 1tsp
- Eggs 4
- Sour cream 1/4 cup
- Superfine Almond Flour 2 cups
- Baking Powder 2tsp

Instructions

1. First, the oven gets preheated to 350 degrees. Grease a 6-cup pan and set it aside. By using a paddle attachment on the blender, beat the butter, cream cheese, and swerve together in a broad mixer bowl until light and fluffy and well blended.

2. Now pour the almond extract and blend thoroughly.

3. The eggs and sour cream are added and then blend well.

4. Mix all the dry ingredients until they are mixed well. Blend the mixture until light and fluffy.

5. Drop the batter into greased pan. Bake it for about 40 minutes until it comes clean with a toothpick inserted into the bottom.

6. Cut slices and freeze individual slices for a quick sweet tooth remedy,

7. Try beating the batter nicely.

8. Just use a Bundt pan for six cups, not the big 10-12 cup pan

Nutrition

Kcal 304, fat 27g, Protein 9g, net carbs 7 g

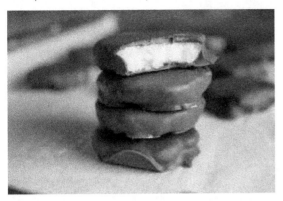

1. Keto Peppermint Patties

Cook time: 5 mins, Servings: 12 patties, Difficulty: easy

Ingredients

- Coconut oil (softened slightly) 0.5 cup
- Coconut cream 2 tbsp.
- Swerve sweetener powdered 0.5 cup
- Peppermint oil /extract 1 - 2 tsp
- Sugar-free chopped dark chocolate 3 ounces.
- Cocoa 0.5 cup

Instructions

1. Put the coconut oil and the coconut cream with each other in a medium bowl until smooth. Whisk together the powdered sweetener tin and 1 tsp of the peppermint extract. If needed, taste and add extra extract.

2. Cover the baking sheet with either parchment or waxed sheets. Dollop onto the paper a heaping tablespoon of the mixture and spread out to a circle of 1 1/2 inches. Repeat the step with the remaining available mixture and freeze for around 2 hours, until solid.

3. Melt together the chocolate and cacao butter in a heatproof bowl positioned over a pan of merely simmering water. Stir until smooth.

4. Drop into the molten chocolate and toss to cover while dealing with one frozen patty at that same time. Remove the extra chocolate with a fork and tap gently on the side of the bowl to remove it.

5. Now put either on a lined tray with parchment paper or wax and leave to set. Repeat the same with the remaining patties.

Nutrition

Kcal 126, fat 13.6g, Protein 0.4g, net carbs 2.9 g

2. Sugar-Free Marshmallows

Cook time: 5 mins, Servings: 10 servings (about 20 marshmallows), Difficulty: easy

Ingredients

- Water 1 cup
- Grass-fed gelatin 2.5 tbsp.
- Swerve sweetener(powdered) 2/3 cup
- Bocha sweet/ xylitol/ allulose 2/3 cup
- Cream of tartar 1/8 tsp
- Pinch salt
- Peppermint extract / vanilla extract 1 tsp

Instructions

1. Line an 8x8 pan with waxed/ parchment paper and grease the paper gently.

2. Mount the stand mixer with the whisk attachment. Through the cup, pour half of the water and brush with the gelatin. When mixing the syrup, let it stand.

3. Mix the rest of the water, the sweeteners, the tartar cream, and the salt in a pot over medium heat. Bring the sweeteners to a boil while stirring.

4. Try bringing the mixture to 237F to 240F temperature using a candy thermometer or an instant-read thermometer. Please remove it from the heat.

5. Set the stand mixer to low and add on the hot syrup slowly down the side of the bowl. Add the extract until all of the syrup is blended in. Adjust the stand mixer to medium-high and beat till the mixture is white, thickened, and lukewarm. It can take 5 to 15 minutes for this.

6. Working fast, pour the blend into the prepared pan dish and smooth the top. Enable 4 to 6 hours until the top is no tackier to the touch.

7. Flip and cut to the appropriate size on a cutting board. If needed, dust with powdered sweetener. Let sit in the air for a day to dry a little, then store in a ziplock container.

Nutrition

Kcal 14, fat 8 g, protein 1.5g, net carbs 0.1 g

3. Keto Sugar-Free Marzipan

Cook time: 30 mins, Servings: 16 servings. Difficulty: easy

Ingredients

- Almond flour 1.5 cups
- Swerve sweetener (Powdered) 1 cup.
- Large egg 1
- Almond extract 2 tsp
- Rosewater 0.5 tsp

Instructions

1. In a food processor, position the blanched almonds and process them until finely ground. Jump to step 2 if the almond meal is used.

2. To mix, introduce the powdered sweetener and pulse. Further, add the egg white, almond extract, and rose water (if consuming) and operate the processor on high until the mixture has become a paste and starts to form a ball.

3. A little extra almond meal is added if the mixture is just too wet. A bit of water, like one teaspoon, is added at a time if the dough seems dry. In texture, it should imitate cookie dough or pastry.

4. Shape into two logs and cover them in plastic wrap tightly. They are usually used for cookies, cake, or candies.

5. Keep the dough tightly packed for a week in the fridge or up to two months in the freezer.

Nutrition

Kcal 65, fat 5.3g, Protein 2.5g, net carbs 2.3 g

4. Keto Rocky Road Fudge

Cook time: 30 mins, Servings: 20 servings, Difficulty: easy

Ingredients

- Homemade marshmallows (sugar-free)3/4
- Heavy whipping cream 1.5 cups
- Bocha sweet 6 tbsp
- Swerve sweetener(powdered) 6 tbsp
- Butter 1/4 cup
- Unsweetened chocolate(chopped) 6 ounces
- Vanilla extract 1 tsp
- Pecan halves 1.5 cups

Instructions

1. Form the marshmallows as per the instructions, but use vanilla extract for replacing the peppermint extract. For drying out properly, these would need to be made a day in advance. Break the marshmallows into 1/2 inch bits and put them on a sheet of cookie lined with parchment paper. Place it in the refrigerator for a minimum of 3 hours.

2. Now line a 9x13 pan with parchment paper.

3. Whisk together both the cream and sweeteners in a broad pan over medium flame. Boil it and then turn the heat down and bring to a simmer for about 30 minutes. Watch closely that it only simmers but does not begin to boil. Small bubbles should be around the edges the entire time.

4. The butter, chopped chocolate, and vanilla extract are added and are withdrawn from the heat before. Sit for 5 minutes until the chocolate and butter have fully melted, then mix until smooth and fluffy.

5. Now the marshmallows and the pecans are to be frozen. Into the prepared pan, distribute the whole mixture evenly. Cool until set, for about three hours, before slicing into squares.

Nutrition Facts

Kcal 155, fat 14.7g, Protein 1.6g, net carbs 2.3 g

5. German Chocolate Truffles

Cook time: 15 mins, Servings: 20 to 24 truffles, Difficulty: easy

Ingredients

- Whipping cream 0.5 cup
- Egg yolks 2
- Swerve sweetener(powdered) 0.5 cup
- Salted butter (sliced into four pieces) 1/4 cup
- Vanilla extract 0.5 tsp
- Unsweetened shredded coconut 3/4 cup
- Pecans (chopped, toasted) 2/3 cup
- Coconut flour 1tsp
- Sugar-free dark chocolate(chopped) 3 ounces
- Cocoa butter / coconut oil 0.5

Instructions

1. First, cover the baking sheet with parchment / waxed paper.

2. Mix the cream, yolk of eggs, sweetener, and butter over a saucepan on medium flame. Cook for approximately 10 minutes, until thickened.

3. Take it off the heat and stir together the vanilla, coconut, and pecans. Sprinkle on the floor with coconut flour and then whisk fast to blend.

4. Let the mixture cool for 10 to 20 minutes, occasionally stirring. Scoop out, tbsp.-sized mounds on the baking sheet when it's still soft but not runny (A small cookie scoop works well). There has to be 20-24 mounds. Freeze it for 1 to 2 hours.

5. Heat up the chocolate and cocoa butter with each other in a heatproof bowl over a pan of gently simmering water till smooth. To extract excess chocolate, dip the refrigerated mounds into the chocolate coating with the help of a fork and then tap the fork tightly against the side of the cup to remove the excess chocolate. Return to waxed paper and leave to set for 10 to 20 minutes.

Nutrition

Kcal 232, fat 22.85g, Protein 2.3g, net carbs 6.49 g

1. No Churn Strawberry Ice Cream

Cook time: 20 mins, Servings: 10 servings, Difficulty: easy

Ingredients

- Strawberries 12 ounces
- Both sweet 1/4 cup
- Fat sour cream 1.5 cups
- Vanilla extract 1tsp
- Heavy cream 1.5 cups
- Swerve sweetener (powdered) 1/3 cup

Instructions

1. Add in a blender/ food processor the strawberries and BochaSweet together. Blend it till almost purified, but some bits are still left.

2. Now whisk the sour cream, vanilla extract, and strawberry mixture together in a mixing bowl until evenly mixed.

3. In yet another big bowl, whip the cream until it maintains rigid peaks with the powdered swerve. Pour the whipped cream gently into the strawberry mixture until there are only a few streaks left.

4. It is moved to an airtight container and freeze for at least 6 hours until stable.

5. Keep it in the refrigerator, so the ice cream can freeze pretty hard. Can introduce a few tablespoons of vodka to the strawberry mixture to offset the frostiness.

Nutrition

Kcal 202, fat 18.6g, Protein 1.7g, net carbs 4.41g

2. Keto Peach Ice Cream

Cook time: 45 mins, Servings: 8 servings, Difficulty: medium

Ingredients

- Ripe peaches (peeled/ sliced) 400 g

- Bocha sweet/ xylitol 1/3 cup

- Lemon juice 1 tbsp

- Heavy whipped cream 1.5 cups

- Unsweetened almond/ hemp milk 0.5 cups

- Swerve sweetener 1/3 cup

- Egg yolks 4

- Salt 1/4 tsp

- Glucomannan powder/xanthan gum 1/2 tsp

- Vodka 2 tbsp

- Vanilla extract 0.5 tsp

Instructions

1. First, put the diced peaches in a bowl and mix with the lemon juice and Bocha Sweet. Wait for 30 minutes to macerate so that juices are released, then mash with a large fork or potato masher. They must be mashed possibly well, but a few tiny bits and pieces are fine.

2. Over an ice bath, position a reasonable bowl and set it aside.

3. Now blend the cream, almond milk, and swerve in a broad saucepan over a medium-low flame. Bring it to a simmer, constantly stirring so that sweetener gets dissolved.

4. Whisk the yolk of eggs with salt in yet another bowl until smooth. Now pour about a half cup of the hot cream into yolks, whisking constantly. After this, slowly pour the mixture of egg yolk back into the saucepan, whisking continually.

5. Keep cooking along with whisking continuously till the mixture on the thermometer reaches 170F or thickens sufficiently to cover a wooden spoon's back. Turn off the heat and pour quickly over the prepared ice bath in the bowl.

6. Let the mashed peach puree cool for 10 minutes, then whisk in. Glucomannan is the whisking medium used. Refrigerate it for duration of 3 hours and up to night-time.

7. Mix in the vanilla extract and vodka and slowly pour into an ice cream maker's canister. Churn, as per instructions of the manufacturer. Then shift it to an airtight container once churned, and freeze for another hour or two until solid enough to scoop.

8. Until fully churned, about 1 1/2 quarts of ice cream are formed from this recipe. And therefore, it could really be split into ten servings.

Nutrition

Kcal 211, fat 18.1g, Protein 2.8g, net carbs 6.5 g

3. Sugar-Free Fudge Pops

Cook time: 5 mins, Servings: 8 popsicles, Difficulty: easy

Ingredients

- Heavy cream 1 cup
- Almond/cashew milk (unsweetened) 1 cup
- Swerve sweetener 1/3 cup
- Cocoa powder (unsweetened) 1/3 cup
- Vanilla extract/ peppermint extract 1tsp
- Xanthan gum 1/4 tsp

Instructions

1. In a saucepan, blend together milk, cream, swerve, and cocoa powder over moderate flame. Boil it and then cook by stirring continuously for one minute.

2. Take off the heat and add on peppermint extract while stirring. To combine, mix with xanthan gum and whisk speedily. Cool it for 10 minutes and then shift into Popsicle molds.

3. Freeze for 1 hour, then press wooden sticks into popsicles and then return back to the freezer (wooden sticks are best to have

stayed in the pops when taken out of the molds). Freeze for about five more hours before solid.

4. Hover under clean hot running water for 30 seconds or so to loosen molds.

Nutrition Facts

Kcal 118, fat 11.2g, Protein 1.44g, net carbs 3.1 g

4. Low Carb Cannoli Ice Cream

Cook time: 10 mins, Servings: 8, Difficulty: easy

Ingredients

- Whipped cream heavy 1 cup
- Swerve sweetener(Powdered) 1/4 cup
- Bochasweet 1/4 cup
- Ricotta cheese 3/4 cup
- Cream cheese 3 ounces
- Vanilla extract 1 tsp
- Lily's chocolate chips (sugar-free) 1/3 cup
- Chopped pistachios (optional) 1/4 cup

Instructions

1. Beat the cream with the Swerve Sweetener in a mixing bowl once it has stiff peaks.

2. Add the ricotta, cream cheese, vanilla extract, and BochaSweet inside a food processor or blender. Mix thoroughly and also have the sweetener dissolved.

3. Fold in the whipped cream with the ricotta mixture. Then fold in the chocolate chips gently.

4. Layer in an airtight jar and chill for 6 to 8 hours until solid.

Nutrition

Kcal 242, fat 20.7g, Protein 5.3g, net carbs 6.4 g

5. Keto Strawberry Lemonade Popsicles

Cook time: 10 mins, Servings: 8, Difficulty: easy

Ingredients

- Sliced strawberries 1 1/4 cup
- A cup of coconut cream 1 1/4 cup
- Squeezed juice of lemon 1/3 cup
- Swerve sweetener(Powdered) 1/3 cup

Instructions

1. Blend the ingredients till fluffy and smooth. Taste the sweetener and change it to your liking.

2. Put over 3-ounces each into Popsicle molds. To release any air trapped bubbles, strike the molds loosely on the counter a few times.

3. Set wooden sticks into the popsicles around 2/3 of the way. (The mixture must be thick enough to hold the sticks in place, but first, freeze the popsicles for 1 hour, then bring them into the sticks).

4. Now freeze it for at least 6- 8 hours.

5. Warm some water in a kettle in order to unmold the popsicles and run it for 5 to 10 seconds outside of the mold, which is to be released. Tug the stick gently in order to remove the Popsicle.

Nutrition

Kcal 117, fat 11.3g, Protein 0.05g, net carbs 2.7 g

6. Sweet Keto Pie Crust

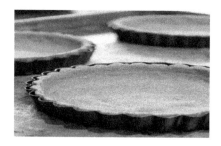

Cook time: 25 mins, Servings: 8, Difficulty: easy

Ingredients

- A cup of almond flour one ¾ cup
- Vanilla/whey protein/ egg white protein powder 1/4 cup
- Erythritol / Swerve(powdered) 1/4 cup
- Egg 1
- Virgin coconut oil/ ghee 2 tbsp.
- Vanilla extract 1 tsp
- Cinnamon 1/2 - 1 tsp
- Pumpkin spice mix 1 tsp
- Food extract (chocolate, almond, etc.,) 1 tsp

Instructions

1. An oven is first preheated to 175 °C/ 350 °F (aided by the fan) or 195 °C/ 380 °F (conventional). All the dry ingredients are blended: the almond flour, whey protein, and powdered Erythritol together.

2. Bring into the coconut oil and egg and process well.

3. Put the dough with a removable bottom in a non-stick pan and press the sides up just to make a "bowl" shape. If required, use a dough roller. Ideally, use a baking sheet as a bottom liner to ensure that the crust does not stick to it.

4. Alternatively, the dough is divided into eight parts and pressed into eight mini tart pans.

5. Position baking paper on top and then weigh the dough down using ceramic baking beans. To avoid the dough from swelling and producing air bubbles, they will be needed, especially if it is a large pie. Locate them inside oven and cook for around 12-15 minutes.

6. Take it out from oven when finished and fill up with your favorite filling (keto lemon flavored curd, chocolate, the whipped cream, creamy textured coconut milk, less-carb custard, some berries, etc.). When not used immediately, let the crust of pie to cool a bit. Keep inside an airtight jar and store at normal temperature for about five days, or freeze for about three months until cooled.

Nutrition

Kcal 181, fat 15.5g, Protein 8.4g, net carbs 2.3 g

7. Low-Carb Cranberry Curd Tarts

Cook time: 30 mins, Serving: 8 tartlets, Difficulty: easy

Ingredients

- A cup of almond flour 2 cups
- Flax meal 4 tbsps.
- Sea salt one pinch
- Butter/ ghee (Unsalted) 2 tbsps.
- Large egg 1
- Low-Carb Cranberry Curd 2 cups
- Heavy whipped cream/coconut cream 1/2 cup

Instructions

1. Get the Low-Carb Cranberry Curd packed. Before using the ad topping, ensure the curd is chilled.

2. Now set the oven to 160 °C/ 320 °F (fan assisted) or 180 °C/ 355 °F to make the pie crust (conventional). Place in a bowl the almond flour, flax meal, and salt and combine to blend. (Note:

For a nut-free substitute, one might use an equal amount of ground sunflower seeds.) Add softened butter (ghee/ coconut oil) and eggs.

3. Just use a spoon or hand to blend dense dough is made. Then use a rolling pin, put the dough between two pieces of clinging film, and roll. Shift the dough into a 9-inch tart pan or into eight different 4-inch pans (without the clinging film).

4. Bake for 8 - 10 mins, until nicely browned and crisped.

5. Take the pie crusts out from the oven before introducing the topping and let it cool slightly.

6. Pour the mixture of cranberry curd into each tartlet (approximately 1/4 cup for each tart).

7. Now whisk the cream (coconut cream) in a bowl till bouncy and fluffy. To top each of the tarts, add a dollop of whipped cream by using a spoon.

8. Place it like an hour in the fridge.

9. Sprinkle with cinnamon as a choice and serve.

10. Store for five days in the fridge.

Nutrition

Kcal 366, fat 33g, Protein 8.9g, net carbs 7.2 g

8. Flaky Keto Pie Crust

Cook time: 20 mins, Serving: 8, Difficulty: easy

Ingredients

- Almond flour 2 cups
- Flax meal 4 tbsps.
- Sea salt pinch
- Unsalted butter/ ghee o/ coconut oil 2 tbsps.
- Large egg 1

Instructions

1. First preheat the oven (fan assisted) to 160 °C/ 320 °F or 180 °C/ 355 °F (conventional). Combine the almond flour, flax flour, and a pinch of salt in a dish.

2. Softened (butter/ghee/coconut oil) and egg are poured.

3. Use the spoon or hand to blend until dense dough is formed.

4. Move it to a 9" (23 cm) greased tart pan, eight separate 4" (10 cm) pans, or four specific 5-inch pans. (Suggestion: It's best to use non-stick pie pans with flexible bottoms. Cover the bottom with a sheet of 9-inch (23 cm) round parchment paper if using a big pie pan.)

5. Force the dough down near the bottom and up the sides to make an edge, using either hand or a small roller. It's safer to use baking beans to weigh down the dough and avoid tiny air bubbles from forming while using a large pie crust. Place it into the oven.

6. Depending on the desired brown color, bake for 8 to 12 minutes, rotating the tray halfway to maintain even cooking. Remove the oven tray and put it on a cooling rack. Remove from the pie pans while cooling down. A sharp blade knife can be used to cut gently the pie crusts when needed.

7. Stock for up to 3 days at normal room temperature in a sealed jar, two weeks to refrigerate, or for three months in the freezer.

Nutrition

Kcal 201, fat 18.1g, Protein 6.8g, net carbs 2.3 g

Conclusion

Thus, on a ketogenic diet, you can eat a large range of delicious and healthy meals. These are not just fats and meats. Vegetables are an integral element of the diet. Perfect snacks for a ketogenic diet include meat, olives, nuts, boiled eggs, cheese, & raw vegetables. For intractable seizures, the keto diet offers safe and reasonably balanced treatment. In view of its long experience, however, much remains uncertain about the diet, including its mechanisms of action, the best care, and the broad reach of its applicability. It is possible to limit several of the side effects of beginning a ketogenic diet. Easing into diet & taking supplements with minerals will help. It can be much simpler to adhere to the ketogenic diet by reading food labels, preparing your meals ahead, and carrying your own food while visiting family and friends.

The ketogenic diet usually has special effects on the body and cells, which may have benefits that go well beyond what almost any diet can offer. The combination of carbohydrate restriction and ketone synthesis reduces insulin rates, stimulates autophagy, enhances mitochondrial chemicals' growth and efficiency, reduces inflammation, and burns fat.

CPSIA information can be obtained
at www.ICGtesting.com
Printed in the USA
BVHW041015150321
602551BV00006B/530